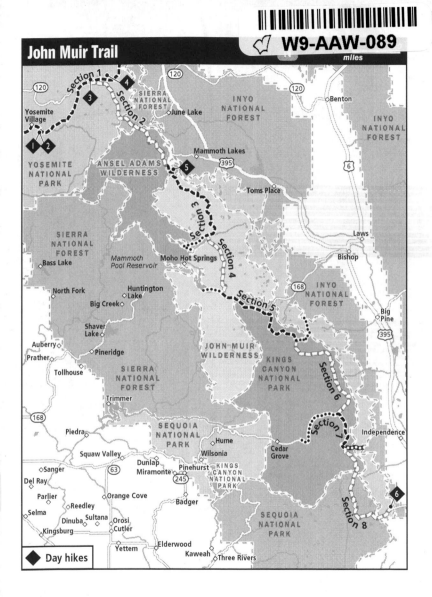

Map Key

Day Hikes

Section Hikes

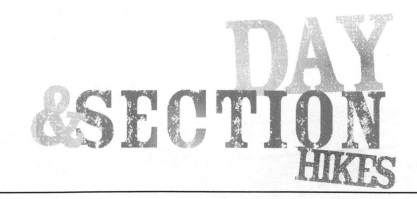

DAY &SECTION HIKES

John Muir Trail

KATHLEEN DODGE

MENASHA RIDGE PRESS

DISCLAIMER

This book is meant only as a guide to the John Muir Trail area and does not guarantee hiker safety in any way—you hike at your own risk. Neither Menasha Ridge Press nor Kathleen Dodge is liable for property loss or damage, personal injury, or death that result in any way from accessing or hiking the trails described in the following pages. Please be aware that hikers have been injured in the John Muir Trail area. Be especially cautious when walking on or near boulders, steep inclines, and drop-offs, and do not attempt to explore terrain that may be beyond your abilities. To help ensure an uneventful hike, please read carefully the introduction to this book, and perhaps get further safety information and guidance from other sources. Familiarize yourself thoroughly with the areas you intend to visit before venturing out. Ask questions, and prepare for the unforeseen. Familiarize yourself with current weather reports, maps of the area you intend to visit, and any relevant park regulations.

Copyright © 2007 by Kathleen Dodge
All rights reserved
Printed in the United States of America
Published by Menasha Ridge Press
Distributed by Publishers Group West
First edition, first printing

Cover and text design by Ian Szymkowiak, Palace Press International, Inc.
Cover photo by John Elk III/Alamy
Maps by Steve Jones, Travis Bryant, and Kathleen Dodge

Library of Congress Cataloging-in-Publication Data

Dodge, Kathleen.
    Day & section hikes: John Muir Trail/Sheri McGregor.—1st ed.
        p. cm.
    Includes index.
    ISBN-13: 978-0-89732-963-7 (alk. paper)
    ISBN-10: 0-89732-963-5 (alk. paper)

    1. Hiking—California—John Muir Trail—Guidebooks. 2. Backpacking—California—
John Muir Trail—Guidebooks. 3. John Muir Trail (Calif.)—Guidebooks. I. Title. II. Title:
Day and section hikes.

    GV199.42.C2D63 2007
    796.5109794—dc22

                                                                    2006100496

Menasha Ridge Press
P.O. Box 43673
Birmingham, AL 35243
www.menasharidge.com

Table of Contents

Section Hikes

Dedication

This book is for my loving and supportive parents. For my dad, who first took me backpacking and inspired my lifelong passion for the outdoors. And to my mom, who packed us frozen Cokes for the car and relished hearing stories of our adventures. It's also for Eric, who allows me the freedom to roam but inspires me to return.

And it would be remiss to not dedicate this book largely to John Muir himself, whose vision, passion, and conservation efforts made these hikes possible.

Acknowledgments

This book never would have been written if Autumn Oden and Marisa Gierlich hadn't been crazy enough to join me on my first John Muir Trail odyssey. Their laughter, patience with my dubious backcountry culinary skills, and unflagging good humor were the backbone of our unforgettable foray. Joining us and providing new food, new jokes, and the occasional new socks was the unparalleled support crew of Kristina Malsberger, Tim Lohnes, Jill Eskes, Paul Burgin, Troy Schaum, and Eric Ople. These hardy souls brought the meaning of friendship to a whole new level. Chocolate cake and red wine under a full moon at 10,000 feet is a birthday never to be forgotten.

This year, I'd like to thank the following souls who joined me for backcountry research: Melanie Leavitt, Chris Baty, Tim Lohnes, and Eric Doherty for being part of the Yosemite send-off crew; Victoria Schlesinger for taking her New York City–honed journalistic skills to the trail and not complaining when the mosquitoes were bigger than the crackers I forgot; Cindy Kopper for keeping the Red's Meadow nights lively; Kelly Perce for braving the road to Vermilion Valley (twice!) and loaning the lifesaving sleeping bag; Ann Cleaveland for grinning for nearly 8 miles uphill despite blisters that would make a mountaineer cry; Jenn Fox and Josh Mangum for ferreting out the best in local produce from fresh currants to toasted pine nuts; Linda Cassell for her high-altitude euphoria that carried us up Whitney even when we ran out of fuel and had dry oatmeal for breakfast. I'd also like to thank Brent Searcy for mapping assistance and the many helpful hikers who gave us rides, shared their beer, and joined us under the stars.

I'd also like to thank the fine folks at Menasha Ridge, particularly Russell Helms, for helping me craft this baby and for believing in the John Muir Trail.

Lastly, I'd like to recognize and acknowledge the many rangers of the Inyo and Sierra national forests. These dedicated men and women are always a delight to meet on the trail and offer a wealth of knowledge. They should be commended for doing their part to help others learn to respect the great outdoors.

—*Kathleen Dodge*

Preface

In *The Mountains of California,* John Muir (1838–1914) writes, "It seemed to me the Sierra should be called not the Nevada, or Snowy Range, but the Range of Light. And after ten years spent in the heart of it, rejoicing and wondering, bathing in its glorious floods of light, seeing the sunbursts of morning among the icy peaks, the noonday radiance on the trees and rocks and snow, the flush of the alpenglow . . . it still seems to me above all others the Range of Light, the most divinely beautiful of all the mountain chains I have ever seen."

Indeed, many would call the Sierra Nevada range one of the finest, most magnificent sights in the world. It seems fitting that the John Muir Trail, which meanders through the very heart of this land that enraptured the man, honors this eccentric and passionate conservationist. Were it not for John Muir's perseverance and dedication to the environment, Yosemite National Park would likely not exist in the pristine state that we find it. Legend holds that John Muir used to climb into the trees during storms to fully embrace the experience. An original tree hugger of sorts.

It was Theodore Solomons (1870–1947), however, who conceived of this classic high route from Yosemite Valley to the top of Mount Whitney (14,495 feet). An early member of the Sierra Club, and the surveyor responsible for naming many of the region's peaks, Solomons reportedly came up with the idea while herding his uncle's sheep at the age of 14. He has since been dubbed the "Father of the John Muir Trail." And in 1915 the Sierra Club broke ground on the trail dedicated to their founder. It took 23 years—and a lot of blood, sweat, and dynamite—for the route to be completed. It's only when you witness firsthand the way the trail snakes over a seemingly impassable chain of unending granite peaks that you can truly appreciate the endeavor. Fittingly, the trail's christening came upon the 100-year anniversary of John Muir's birth. While born in Scotland and not setting foot in Yosemite until he was 30 years old, Muir was a vastly successful crusader in saving California's wild lands.

The pull of the Range of Light remains strong: These days more than 800 hikers are drawn each year to complete the John Muir Trail. They come for different reasons, from different places, and with different expectations, but they all come away affected by their journey. Stretching out over more than 200 glorious miles between Yosemite and Mount Whitney, the trail climbs over ten high-altitude passes (over half of which are above 11,000 feet) and includes an ascent of the highest point in the lower 48 states. By all accounts, the trail is a big, beefy wilderness experience worthy of the accolades heaped upon it. Unlike some long trails, the John Muir Trail is a true wilderness experience: One needn't cross roads, see cars, or take a hot shower for the entire stretch. Resupplies must be mailed or packed in to remote locations, and there isn't cell phone coverage for miles and miles. For much of the way, the JMT and Pacific Crest Trail (a 2,650-mile route from Canada to Mexico, originally blazed in 1930) mirror each other, and this stretch is considered the most spectacular of the PCT's long journey.

Without a doubt, tackling the John Muir Trail in one fell swoop is a worthy quest for any hiker. There is a sense of accomplishment and journey that prevails when you travel more than 220 miles from point to point without reentering civilization. It makes the hike feel that much more remote and the adventure that much more epic.

For many, however, hiking the John Muir Trail is a dream that needs to be realized over the course of several months or years. Not everyone has the vacation time, desire, or physical rigor to withstand three or more weeks in the backcountry. Yet that certainly doesn't mean you can't enjoy this glorious stretch of country. For this reason, we've designed a book to allow hikers to get a taste of the trail via various day hikes and to complete the trail via a series of different sections that can be combined to eventually traverse the route in its entirety. We've divided the sections into the shortest possible routes given the remote nature of the trail, and we've selected the most accessible entry and exit points to allow you to plan your journey. We've also chosen routes that are fantastic backcountry journeys in their own right. Thru-hikers will find the sections a useful resource for friends who want to join them on shorter legs of their journey.

Whatever the length of your stay, may you come away from your experience as John Muir did when he wrote *My First Summer in the Sierra* in 1911, proclaiming "Exhilarated with the mountain air, I feel like shouting this morning with excess of wild animal joy!"

Top Hikes Lists

Most Scenic Hikes

All are scenic, but especially Florence Lake to South Lake.

Most Difficult Hikes

Vermilion Valley to Florence Lake (page 100)

Onion Valley to Mount Whitney (page 138)

Easiest Hikes

Lyell Canyon (page 42)

Devils Postpile and Rainbow Falls (page 48)

Red's Meadow to Vermilion Valley (page 88)

Best-maintained Trails

All are well maintained.

Best for Solitude

Florence Lake to South Lake (page 110)

Best for Children

Cathedral Lakes (page 38)

Lyell Canyon (page 42)

Devils Postpile and Rainbow Falls (page 48)

Best Wildflower Hikes

You can't go wrong with any of these hikes.

Best Wildlife Hikes

Roads End to Onion Valley (page 130)

Steep Hikes

All are steep, but especially the following:

Mount Whitney (page 56)

Onion Valley to Mount Whitney (page 138)

Flat Hikes

Lyell Canyon (page 42)

Introduction

How to Use This Guidebook

THIS GUIDE breaks the John Muir Trail, traditionally a two- to four-week journey, into manageable day and section hikes. These can be used to conquer the trail in bits or combined into one full thru-hike. The sections can also be used to have other hikers join you, allow for resupplying of food and equipment, and offer entry and exit points to your hike.

THE OVERVIEW MAP AND OVERVIEW-MAP KEY

Use the overview map on the inside front cover to assess the exact locations of each hike's primary trailhead. Each hike's number appears on the overview map, on the map key facing the overview map, and in the table of contents. As you flip through the book, a hike's full profile is easy to locate by watching for the hike number at the top of each page. A map legend that details the symbols found on trail maps appears on the inside back cover.

TRAIL MAPS

Each hike contains a detailed map that shows the trailhead, the route, significant features, facilities, and topographic landmarks such as creeks, overlooks, and peaks. The author gathered map data by carrying a GPS unit (Garmin eTrex Legend) while hiking. This data was downloaded into a digital mapping program (DeLorme's TopoUSA) and processed by expert cartographers to produce the highly accurate maps found in this book. Each trailhead's GPS coordinates are included with each profile (see page 2).

ELEVATION PROFILES

Corresponding directly to the trail map, each hike contains a detailed elevation profile. The elevation profile provides a quick look at the trail from the side, enabling you to visualize how the trail rises and falls. Note the number of feet between each tick mark on the vertical axis (the height scale). To avoid making flat hikes look steep and steep hikes appear flat, different height scales are used throughout the book to provide an accurate image of the hike's climbing difficulty.

GPS TRAILHEAD COORDINATES

To collect accurate map data, each trail was hiked with a handheld GPS unit (Garmin eTrex Legend). In addition to rendering a highly specific trail outline, this book also includes the GPS coordinates for each trailhead in two formats: UTM (Universal Transverse Mercator) and latitude–longitude.

Topographic maps show latitude–longitude as well as UTM grid lines. Known as UTM coordinates, the numbers index a specific point using a grid method. The survey datum used to arrive at the coordinates in this book is WGS84 (versus NAD27 or WGS83). For readers who own a GPS unit, whether handheld or onboard a vehicle, the latitude–longitude or UTM coordinates provided at the end of each hike may be entered into the GPS unit. Just make sure your GPS unit is set to navigate using WGS84 datum. Now you can navigate directly to the trailhead.

Most trailheads, which begin in parking areas, can be reached by car, but some hikes still require a short walk to reach the trailhead from a parking area. In those cases, a handheld unit is necessary to continue the GPS navigation process. That said, however, readers can easily access all trailheads in this book by using the directions given, the overview map, and the trail map, which shows at least one major road leading into the area. But for those who enjoy using the latest GPS technology to navigate, the necessary data has been provided. A brief explanation of the UTM and latitude–longitude coordinates from the Vernal and Nevada Falls hike (page 26) follows.

UTM zone (WGS84)	11S
Easting	0274558
Northing	4179230
Latitude	N 37°43'57.31"
Longitude	W 119°33'31.47"

The UTM zone number **11** refers to one of the 60 vertical zones of the UTM projection, each of which is 6 degrees wide. The UTM zone letter **S** refers to one of the 20 horizontal zones that span from 80 degrees South to 84 degrees North. The easting number **0274558** indicates in meters how far east or west a point is from the central meridian of the zone. Increasing easting coordinates on a topo map or on your GPS screen indicate that you are moving east; decreasing easting coordinates indicate you are moving west. The northing number **4179230** references in meters how far you are from the equator. Above and below the equator, increasing northing coordinates indicate you are traveling north; decreasing northing coordinates indicate you are traveling south.

Latitude–longitude coordinates tell you where you are by locating a point west (longitude) of the 0° meridian line that passes through Greenwich, England, and north or south of the 0° (latitude) line that belts the earth (the equator).

To learn more about how to enhance your outdoor experiences with GPS technology, refer to *GPS Outdoors: A Practical Guide for Outdoor Enthusiasts* (Menasha Ridge Press).

The Hike Narrative

In addition to maps, each hike profile contains a concise but informative narrative of the hike from beginning to end. This descriptive text is enhanced with at-a-glance ratings and information, GPS-based trailhead coordinates, and accurate driving directions that lead you from a major road to the parking area most convenient to the trailhead.

At the top of the section for each hike is a box that allows the hiker quick access to pertinent information: quality of scenery, condition of trail, appropriateness for children, difficulty of hike, quality of solitude expected, hike distance, approximate time of hike, and outstanding highlights of the trip. The first five categories are rated using a five-star system. An example follows:

1 Vernal and Nevada Falls

SCENERY: ☆ ☆ ☆ ☆ ☆
TRAIL CONDITION: ☆ ☆ ☆ ☆
CHILDREN: ☆ ☆ ☆
DIFFICULTY: ☆ ☆ ☆
SOLITUDE: ☆

DISTANCE: *7 miles*
HIKING TIME: *4–6 hours*
OUTSTANDING FEATURES: *Vernal Falls, Nevada Falls, Emerald Pool, Silver Apron, Clark Point, sweeping views of the valley*

The five stars indicate that the scenery is very picturesque. The trail condition is very good (one star would mean the trail is likely to be muddy, rocky, overgrown, or otherwise compromised). The hike is doable for able-bodied children (a one-star rating would denote that only the most gung ho and physically fit children should go). The three stars in the fourth category indicate that the hike is moderately difficult (five stars for difficulty would be strenuous). Finally, you can expect to encounter quite a few people on the trail (with five stars you may well be alone on your way up the trail).

Distances given are absolute, but hiking times are estimated for an average hiking speed of 2 to 3 miles per hour, with time built in for pauses at overlooks and brief rests. Overnight-hiking times account for the effort of carrying a backpack.

Following each box is a brief italicized description of the hike. A more detailed account follows in which trail junctions, stream crossings, and trailside features are noted along with their distance from the trailhead. Flip through the book, read the descriptions, and choose a hike that appeals to you.

Weather

It has been said that the Sierra Nevada range enjoys the best weather of any chain of mountains in the world. The hiking season, while short due to lingering snowpack, is characterized by clear sunny days with only the occasional summer afternoon thunderstorm. But weather conditions in mountain systems, as a general rule, are unpredictable and quick to change without warning. When preparing for a hike in the Sierra Nevada, it is still best to expect the unexpected; snow in August and blistering heat in the fall are not unheard of. It's vital that you prepare for a variety of elements: rain, sun, wind, and chill. Much of the trail is above 10,000 feet, and altitude plays a role in warmth as well. As a rule of thumb, the temperature decreases about 3 degrees with every 1,000 feet of elevation gained.

That said, you can rely on certain patterns to help plan your trip. Depending on the winter snowfall, hiking can begin as early as May or as late as July. Spring brings a gorgeous display of wildflowers, vernal pools, a greater chance of rain, more difficult river crossings, fewer crowds than the summer, and abundant snowfields. Summer brings sunshine-filled views, mosquitoes, more crowds, warm nights, longer days, and very little rain save for the afternoon thunderstorm. Fall brings autumnal color displays as the leaves change, fewer crowds, virtually no bugs, and cooler, earlier nightfall. Winter brings short days, snowfall, and the need for skis or snowshoes. Winter camping in the high Sierra requires experience and equipment that is not covered in this guidebook. The first snows of winter usually arrive in October and November, and snow can fall intermittently through May.

Average Temperature (Fahrenheit) by Month

	Jan	Feb	Mar	Apr	May	Jun
High	47	55	58	65	71	80
Low	25	26	30	34	39	46
Rainfall	6.4"	6.6"	5.9"	3.3"	1.5"	0.5"

	Jul	Aug	Sep	Oct	Nov	Dec
High	89	89	82	72	57	49
Low	50	50	48	39	30	26
Rainfall	0.3"	0.1"	0.6"	1.7"	3.5"	7.1"

Water

How much is enough? Well, one simple physiological fact should convince you to err on the side of excess when deciding how much water to pack: A hiker working hard in 90-degree heat needs approximately 10 quarts of fluid per day. That's 2.5 gallons— 12 large water bottles or 16 small ones. In other words, pack along one or two bottles even for short hikes.

For longer trips there's no way to carry enough water, and hikers and backpackers will need to treat their drinking water to make it safe. There are three ways to do so: boiling, purification filters, and chemical treatment procedures. Bringing water to a rapid boil for one minute will kill all harmful microorganisms. However, boiling water on the trail on a hot day is not always the most efficient or palatable option or the best use of fuel. Most hikers will pack a purification filter. There are a variety of lightweight portable purifiers on the market, but the ones with ceramic filters are the safest. It's also a good idea to pack along the slightly distasteful tetraglycine-hydroperiodide or chlorine tablets to debug water (sold under the names Potable Aqua, Coughlan's, and others). In the case of filter failure, these tablets are invaluable, and adding a little tasty powdered beverage mix can help mask the chemical flavor.

Probably the most common waterborne "bug" that hikers face is giardia, which may not hit until one to four weeks after ingestion. It will have you living in the bathroom, passing noxious rotten-egg gas, vomiting, and shivering with chills. Other parasites to worry about include E. coli and cryptosporidium, both of which are harder to kill than giardia.

Happily, streams, creeks, and lakes are readily available nearly everywhere in the Sierra Nevada. And while we don't recommend drinking straight from the source, you can still enjoy cold, refreshing alpine water that has been filtered. But please don't eat the yellow snow!

Clothing

Packing for a hike is a bit of a science—you want to have enough gear to be prepared for anything while not carrying so much that you feel like a pack mule. The length and season of your hike will largely guide your decisions, but the following information can help you prepare. We've also included a general packing list for overnight trips that you can use as a guideline for your own adventures.

There is a wide variety of clothing from which to choose. Basically, use common sense and be prepared for anything. If all you have are cotton clothes when a sudden rainstorm comes along, you'll be miserable, especially in cooler weather. It's a good idea to bring quick-drying synthetic fabrics (polypropylene, Capilene, Thermax, and the like), and to layer your clothes so that you can monitor your temperature as the weather shifts.

Fleece and goose down are excellent lightweight warmth providers. Goose down is particularly wonderful for its featherlight heavy-duty insulation, but take care not to get it wet, as it takes a long time to dry. A down vest is useful to keep your core warm; it won't take up much room in your pack and makes an excellent pillow when stuffed into a thin pillowcase. A hat and gloves are essential for high altitude nights—often freezing even in the summer.

Raingear is a must as thunderstorms can come on suddenly and soak you to the bone. Getting wet opens the door to hypothermia. A lightweight rain jacket (be sure it's rainproof and not simply water resistant!) that you can layer over other clothes is recommended. In addition to the raingear that you wear, it's useful to have a thin plastic tarp that can double as a ground cloth for your tent and a makeshift shelter in a storm.

Much of the trail is at high elevation in exposed areas above treeline. A good hat and sunscreen are crucial to protect your face from the bright sun. The white granite and pumice trail can also be murder on your eyes without sunglasses.

During particularly buggy seasons, a mosquito head net can be a saving grace. While not the most fashion forward, these can make the difference between a miserable day and an enjoyable hike.

Footwear is a great debate among hikers. Generally speaking, waterproof boots with ankle support are widely regarded as your safest option for warmth, protection, and dependability. Some argue, however, that the weight of hefty boots is unnecessarily hard on the knees. Lightweight trail-running shoes provide enough support and durability for many, but they are not usually waterproof. Around camp, a pair of lightweight, open slip-on shoes (such as Crocs) is an excellent choice, allowing for comfort as well as the wearing of socks during chilly nights. Your camp shoes should be able to double as river-crossing shoes in the early season. A good pair of wool socks, warm even when wet, paired with silk or synthetic sock liners, is an excellent safeguard against blisters, which can ruin your trip. See the packing list in Appendix A for details.

Packing Tips

· Wrap duct tape around your water bottle for lightweight efficiency.

· Line your sleeping-bag stuff sack with a garbage bag.

· Bend tent poles from the middle to keep tension on the spring cord even while contracted, extending the life of your tent poles.

The Ten Essentials

One of the first rules of hiking is to be prepared for anything. The simplest way to be prepared is to carry the "Ten Essentials." In addition to carrying the items listed below, you need to know how to use them, especially navigation items. Always consider worst-case scenarios like getting lost, hiking back in the dark, broken gear (for example, a broken hip strap on your pack or a water filter getting plugged), twisting an ankle, or a brutal thunderstorm. The items listed below don't cost a lot of money, don't take up much room in a pack, and don't weigh much, but they might just save your life.

WATER: durable bottles, and water treatment such as iodine and a filter

MAP: preferably a topo map and a trail map with a route description

COMPASS: a high-quality compass

FIRST-AID KIT: a good-quality kit including first-aid instructions

KNIFE: a multitool device with pliers is best

LIGHT: flashlight or headlamp with extra bulbs and batteries

FIRE: windproof matches or lighter and fire starter

EXTRA FOOD: you should always have some left in your pack after a hike

EXTRA CLOTHES: rain protection, warm layers, gloves, warm hat

SUN PROTECTION: sunglasses, lip balm, sunblock, sun hat

Hiking with Children

No one is too young for a hike in the outdoors. Be mindful, though. Flat, short, and shaded trails are best with an infant. Toddlers who have not quite mastered walking can still tag along, riding on an adult's back in a child carrier. Use common sense to judge a child's capacity to hike a particular trail, and always factor in that the child will tire quickly and need to be carried. A list of hikes suitable for children is provided on page xiv.

Many children enjoy longer backpacking trips, and this can be a wonderful way to introduce your kids to the joys of sleeping under the stars. However, in order to ensure a fun trip for everyone, you need to prepare accordingly. In general, young children (5 to 7) should never carry more than 5 to 10 percent of their body weight, and older kids (8 to 12) shouldn't graduate past 25 percent of their weight. Start out with short distances and include frequent water breaks, swimming stops, and snacks as your kids become accustomed to the process.

General Safety

Despite what creepy movies may have led you to believe, you'll be much safer in the woods than in most urban areas of the country. No doubt, potentially dangerous situations can occur outdoors, but as long as you use sound judgment and prepare yourself before hitting the trail, you should enjoy a safe and happy backcountry hike. Here are a few tips to help guide your preparation.

- **RECOGNIZE THE SIGNS OF ALTITUDE SICKNESS.** With much of the John Muir Trail above treeline, it is normal to feel mild effects of the altitude as shortness of breath, slight headache, loss of appetite, and difficulty sleeping as you ascend over 6,000 feet. These symptoms should dissipate as you acclimate, and you should not continue gaining altitude if they remain. At the onset of vomiting, disorientation, or loss of coordination, it's vital that you descend 2,000 to 3,000 feet immediately. If altitude sickness remains untreated, you risk developing HAPE (high-altitude pulmonary edema), an extremely dangerous and life-threatening condition. This is not the kind of sickness to "push through." The best way to prevent altitude sickness is to ascend gradually, ideally no more than 1,000 feet per day when you're above 10,000 feet. Drink plenty of water, eat high-carb foods, and avoid fat. See Appendix B for a list of items to take in your first-aid kit.

- **KNOW WHAT PRECAUTIONS TO TAKE IN THE EVENT OF AN ELECTRICAL STORM.** When lightning is striking, get away from open water, tent poles, tall trees, exposed ground, metal conductors, and single trees. If you are in an exposed area, move to a valley or ravine. If you are in a forested area, seek out stands of small trees. Sit or stand on a ground cover or sleeping pad to insulate yourself from ground conduction.

- **ALWAYS CARRY FOOD AND WATER,** whether you are planning to go overnight or not. Food will give you energy, help keep you warm, and sustain you in an emergency situation until help arrives. You never know if you will have a stream nearby when you become thirsty. Bring potable water or treat water before drinking it from a stream. Boil or filter all found water before drinking it.

- **STAY ON DESIGNATED TRAILS.** Most hikers get lost when they leave the path. Even on the most clearly marked trails, there is usually a point where you have to stop and consider which direction to head. If you become disoriented, don't panic. As soon as you think you may be off-track, stop, assess your current direction, and then retrace your steps back to the point where you went awry. Using a map, a compass, and this book, and keeping in mind what you have passed thus far, reorient yourself and trust your judgment on which way to continue. Should you become completely lost and have no idea of how to return to the trailhead, remaining in place along the trail and waiting for help is most often the best option for adults and always the best option for children.

- **BE ESPECIALLY CAREFUL WHEN CROSSING STREAMS.** Whether you are fording the stream or crossing on a log, make every step count. If you have any doubt about maintaining your balance on a foot log, go ahead and ford the stream instead. When fording a stream, use a trekking pole or stout stick for balance and face upstream as you cross. If a stream seems too deep to ford, turn back. Whatever is on the other side is not worth risking your life.

- **BE CAREFUL AT OVERLOOKS.** While these areas may provide spectacular views, they are potentially hazardous. Stay back from the edge of outcrops and be absolutely sure of your footing; a misstep can mean a nasty and possibly fatal fall.

- **STANDING DEAD TREES AND STORM-DAMAGED LIVING TREES** pose a real hazard to hikers and tent campers. These trees may have loose or broken limbs that could fall at any time. When choosing a spot to rest or a backcountry campsite, look up.

- **KNOW THE SYMPTOMS OF HYPOTHERMIA.** Shivering and forgetfulness are the two most common indicators of this insipid killer. Hypothermia can occur at any elevation, even in the summer, especially when the hiker is wearing lightweight cotton clothing. If symptoms arise, get the victim shelter, hot liquids, and dry clothes or a dry sleeping bag.

- **TAKE ALONG YOUR BRAIN.** A cool, calculating mind is the single most important piece of equipment you'll ever need on the trail. Think before you act. Watch your step. Plan ahead. Avoiding accidents before they happen is the best recipe for a rewarding and relaxing hike.

- **ASK QUESTIONS.** Forest rangers are there to help. It's a lot easier to gain advice beforehand and avoid a mishap away from civilization, where finding help may be difficult. Use your head out there and treat the place as if it were your own backyard. After all, it is your national forest.

Animal and Plant Hazards

Ticks

Ticks like to hang out in the brush that grows along trails. Hot summer months seem to explode their numbers, but you should be tick-aware during all months of the year. Ticks, which are arthropods and not insects, need a host to feast on in order to reproduce. The ticks that light onto you while hiking will be very small, sometimes so tiny that you won't be able to spot them. Primarily of two varieties, deer ticks and dog ticks, both need a few hours of actual attachment before they can transmit any disease they may harbor. Ticks may settle in shoes,

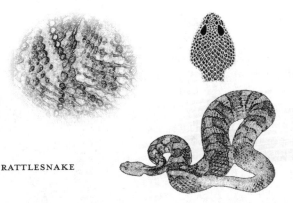

RATTLESNAKE

socks, and hats, and may take several hours to actually latch on. The best strategy is to visually check every half-hour or so while hiking, do a thorough check before you get in the car, and then, when you take a posthike shower, do an even more thorough check of your entire body. Ticks that haven't attached are easily removed, but not easily killed. If you pick off a tick in the woods, just toss it aside. If you find one on your body at home, dispatch it and then send it down the toilet. For ticks that have embedded, removal with tweezers is best.

SNAKES

It is common to spend an entire summer hiking the John Muir Trail and never see a single snake. They tend to be shy creatures that flee at the first sign of human presence. For the most part, the Sierra's snakes are of the small, harmless gopher and garter variety. The western rattlesnake is the only venomous snake to call the region home and usually only at elevations of 6,000 feet or below. As their name suggests, these fellows normally give a distinctive warning before striking, and their strike isn't always accompanied by a bite. There is no need to fear these helpful animals that keep the rodent population down. If you are lucky enough to see one sunning itself on the trail, simply back up and give it a wide berth.

Poison Oak

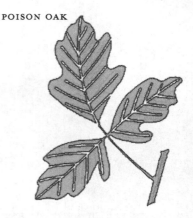

Recognizing, and avoiding, poison oak is the most effective way to prevent the painful, itchy rashes associated with this common California plant. Poison oak occurs at lower elevations of 5,000 feet or below as either a climbing vine or leafy shrub with three leaflets. The Boy Scouts handily proclaim, "Leaves of three, let it be." In the autumn, the leaves turn a shiny red that makes it easy to avoid, but it can blend in more easily in the spring and summer. Urushiol, the oil in the sap of these plants, is responsible for the rash. Usually within 12 to 14 hours of exposure (but sometimes much later), raised lines and/or blisters will appear, accompanied by a terrible itch. Refrain from scratching because bacteria under fingernails can cause infection, and you will spread the rash to other parts of your body. Wash and dry the rash thoroughly, applying a calamine lotion or other product to help dry the rash. If itching or blistering is severe, seek medical attention. Remember that oil-contaminated clothes, pets, or hiking gear can easily cause an irritating rash on you or someone else, so wash not only any exposed parts of your body but also clothes, gear, and pets.

Mosquitoes

Although it's not a common occurrence, individuals can become infected with the West Nile virus by being bitten by an infected mosquito. Culex mosquitoes, the primary variety that can transmit West Nile virus to humans, thrive in urban rather than natural areas. They lay their eggs in stagnant water and can breed in any standing water that remains for more than five days. Most people infected with West Nile virus have no symptoms of illness, but some may become ill, usually 3 to 15 days after being bitten.

While West Nile virus is not a common threat in the Sierra Nevada backcountry, mosquitoes can be a fearsome annoyance on their own. In late spring and summer, and anytime you expect mosquitoes to be buzzing around, you may want to wear protective clothing, such as long sleeves, long pants, head nets, and socks. Loose-fitting, light-colored clothing is best. Spray clothing with insect repellent. Remember to follow the instructions on the repellent and to take extra care with children.

Black Bears

Black bears, which are really often reddish or brown, are the only bear species currently found in California. Unlike unpredictable and fearsome grizzly bears, black bears are North America's smallest bear (although still weighing in at 300 to 400 pounds!) and are more interested in your food than anything else. It is extremely rare for a black bear to act aggressively toward humans, and it is almost always due to human provocation. That's not to say that black bears can't be destructive. They will go to great lengths to secure a free meal—everything from tearing the door off a car to raiding a carelessly maintained camp. With the great numbers of snack-supplying hikers, local bears have become more and more clever; it is no longer a viable option to hang your food, as bears have learned to undo your handiwork. Bear-proof food containers are as necessary as wilderness permits for overnight backcountry adventures along the John Muir Trail. These can be purchased at nearly every California camping-supply store or rented from the Forest Service when you pick up your permit. These canisters are as much to protect the bears as they are your food. Bears who develop a taste for sugary, salty, high-calorie human food are those who are most likely to harass campers in search of their next fix. Park rangers will fine campers without bear canisters and escort them out of the park. You will be doing everybody a favor by properly storing your food (and scented toiletries that could be mistaken for food). If you do see a bear on the trail or in your camp, it is best to back away slowly while shouting loudly and making noise to scare off the animal. Never try to wrestle food away from a bear, and do not get between a mother and her cub.

Mountain Lions

Mountain lions are the largest cats found in North America, but your chances of seeing one are extremely small (most hikers are content to simply look for the cat's four-toed print on the trail). Sometimes called cougars or pumas, they are shy, solitary creatures that hunt (mostly deer) alone and are masters at camouflage with their tawny coats and preference for wooded cover. They can grow up to eight feet in length, including their distinctively long tails. In the unlikely instance that you should come across a mountain lion, you should make eye contact, try to appear larger by spreading your arms, and make noise. Do not run from a mountain lion, as this may trigger its natural instinct to chase you.

Tips for Enjoying the John Muir Trail

The John Muir Trail offers an abundance of pleasures great and small. In the high altitude, you soar above the treeline with wide granite expanses and endless views. In lower elevations, relish the rich diversity of flora in sunny meadows and shady forest thickets. And throughout, find a range of lakes, streams, rivers, and distinct ecosystems. Enjoy them all! In addition, the following tips will make your visit enjoyable and rewarding.

- **TAKE YOUR TIME ALONG THE TRAILS.** Pace yourself. Stop and smell the wildflowers. Peer into a clear mountain stream for rainbow trout. Don't miss the trees for the forest. Shorter hikes allow you to stop and linger more than long hikes. Something about staring at the front end of a 10-mile trek naturally pushes you to speed up. That said, take close notice of the elevation maps that accompany each hike. If you see many ups and down over large altitude changes, you'll obviously need more time. Inevitably you'll finish some of the "hike times" long before or after what is suggested. Nevertheless, leave yourself plenty of time for those moments when you simply feel like stopping and taking it all in.

• **TRY TO HIKE DURING THE WEEK,** and avoid the traditional holidays if possible. (Of course, this is an ideal situation—we can't always schedule our free time when we want.) Trails that are packed in the summer are often clear during the colder months. If you are hiking on a busy day, go early in the morning; it'll enhance your chances of seeing wildlife.

Wilderness Permits

The John Muir Trail passes through several different, and sometimes overlapping, protected backcountry areas: Yosemite, Kings Canyon and Sequoia national parks, Inyo and Sierra national forests (including the John Muir and Ansel Adams wilderness areas), and Devils Postpile National Monument. Each of these designations carries its own rules, regulations, and permit systems. As a simple rule of thumb, national parks are maintained in the interest of conservation and generally carry a larger degree of wilderness protection than national-forest land, which is ordained for "multiple use" and includes everything from cattle grazing to hunting to recreation. The Wilderness Act, a designation enacted in 1964, establishes the highest degree of protection for the country's most pristine and fragile lands. Wilderness areas are generally free from commercial activity, roads, and motorized activity.

Permits and trail quotes vary from trailhead to trailhead. Normally about 60 percent of trailhead permits are reserved with the remaining 40 percent set aside for walk-ins. It's worth noting, however, that in busy areas like Yosemite these nonreserved permits disappear quickly as well. Day hikes do not normally require a permit.

The only exception to this rule is Mount Whitney, where interest and crowds have necessitated that a lottery system for permits be introduced. You will find the appropriate permit information for each hike at the end of the detailed description.

Those seeking to thru-hike the John Muir Trail in its entirety on one trip must also apply for a permit. The first decision you need to make is whether to head south or north. Traditionally, hikers started south and headed north, losing more than 4,000 feet overall en route to Yosemite Valley. Starting at Mount Whitney, however, before you are acclimated and conditioned can be a rather daunting and brutal way to begin your adventure. Today more and more hikers are doing southbound journeys, and this is what we heartily recommend. The terrain out of Yosemite, while certainly not easy, is far gentler and at lower elevation, allowing you to gradually get used to the altitude and miles.

To begin your trip in Yosemite, make a reservation as far in advance as possible; reservations are accepted from 2 days to up to 24 weeks in advance of your trip. You can reserve by calling the Yosemite Wilderness Center at (209) 372-0740 (8:30 a.m. to 4:30 p.m., Monday through Friday) or by reserving online at www.**yosemite.org/ visitor/wild.html.** You can also make reservations by sending mail to Wilderness Reservations, Yosemite Association, P.O. Box 545, Yosemite, CA 95389. For any of these methods, you will need to provide the following information:

- Your name
- Address
- Daytime phone number
- Number of people in the party
- Method of travel (foot)
- Number of stock (if applicable)
- Start and end dates
- Entry and exit trailheads (Happy Isles entry, Whitney Portal exit)

- Principal destination (John Muir Trail)
- Credit-card number and expiration date, money order, or check for a nonrefundable $5-per-person processing fee.

You could also hope for a walk-in permit at the Yosemite Valley Wilderness Center, located in Yosemite Village next to the post office (open seasonally from 9 a.m. to 5 p.m.). However, this is a risky proposition, given all the preparation needed for the trip. To begin your trip in Whitney Portal and head north, the process is a bit different. One hundred percent of all permits are reserved in advance due to the high numbers who want to spend time in the Whitney Zone (the area stretching from Lone Pine Lake to Crabtree Meadow). To make reservations, contact the Inyo National Forest Wilderness Permit Reservation Office (351 Pacu Lane, Suite 200, Bishop, CA 93514). It is open daily 8 a.m. to 4:30 p.m., June 1 to October 1, and Monday through Friday during the rest of the year. You can reserve over the phone at (760) 873-2483, by fax at (760) 873-2484, or by mail. To begin your hike, you must pick up your permit at the Eastern Sierra InterAgency Visitor Center (at the junction of US 395 and CA 136), 2 miles south of Lone Pine Lake. Office hours are 8 a.m. to 5 p.m.; (760) 876-6200. Walk-in permits for unclaimed reservations are available starting at 11 a.m. on the day before your entry date.

Backcountry Advice

In addition to the all-important adages "Pack it in, pack it out," "Take only pictures, leave only footprints," and "Leave no trace," there are a few other important things to know about the Sierra Nevada backcountry.

Open fires are permitted only below 10,000 feet. Below 10,000 feet, firewood should be collected only from downed trees and sticks near your campsite.

Solid human waste must be buried in a hole at least 3 inches deep and at least 200 feet away from trails and water sources; a trowel is basic backpacking equipment. In the Whitney Zone, rangers are encouraging everyone to pack out their human waste with their garbage. You can pick up a "wag bag" at Whitney Portal and dispose of it there as well.

Storing your food properly is essential. Clever Sierra Nevada bears have made hanging food obsolete, and bear-proof canisters are a necessity. Campers without them will be fined by rangers and asked to leave the park. Some areas on the trail have bear-proof boxes available in popular camping areas, but you should still carry your own food-storage system.

Trail Etiquette

Whether you're on a city, county, state, or national park trail, always remember that great care and resources (from nature as well as from your tax dollars) have gone into creating these trails. Treat the trail, wildlife, and fellow hikers with respect.

- **HIKE ON OPEN TRAILS ONLY.** Respect trail and road closures (ask if not sure), avoid possible trespassing on private land, and obtain all permits and authorization as required. Also, leave gates as you found them or as marked.

- **LEAVE ONLY FOOTPRINTS.** Be sensitive to the ground beneath you. This also means staying on the existing trail and not blazing any new trails. Be sure to pack out what you pack in. No one likes to see the trash someone else has left behind.

- **NEVER SPOOK ANIMALS.** An unannounced approach, a sudden movement, or a loud noise startles most animals. A surprised animal can be dangerous to you, to others, and to themselves. Give them plenty of space. If you encounter a pack mule or horse train, step off the trail as best you can and allow them to pass. Large backpacks can frighten these animals.

- **PLAN AHEAD.** Know your equipment, your ability, and the area in which you are hiking—and prepare accordingly. Be self-sufficient at all times; carry necessary supplies for changes in weather or other conditions. A well-executed trip is a satisfaction to you and to others.

- **BE COURTEOUS TO THOSE YOU MEET ON YOUR HIKE.**

Resupplying on the Trail

Each section hike provides detailed information on how to access the trail. Two or three sections could also be combined for hikers looking for a longer backcountry experience. Depending on whether you're driving to the trailhead, being picked up by friends, hitch-hiking, or relying on public transit may determine which trailheads are best for you.

If you are planning to thru-hike the trail or are linking together several sections, then resupplying your food is an important consideration. We've listed several options below that allow you to enjoy your wilderness experience without starving to death. Another option is to have friends join you for part of the trail and bring you food. The one option that has gained some notoriety that we **don't** recommend is having friends leave food caches in bear boxes for you to pick up en route. The problem with this plan is that your food takes up valuable space in bear boxes for days. And often hikers abandon their trail plans and their food rots in the bear boxes, leaving a mess for rangers to clean up.

TUOLUMNE MEADOWS

You can mail food to the post office in Tuolumne Meadows. It needs to be picked up between 8 a.m. and 5:30 p.m. and will be kept for only 10 days (per United States Postal Service regulations). Mail to:

> [Your name]
> General Delivery
> Tuolumne Meadows Station
> Yosemite National Park, CA 95389

RED'S MEADOW

Between June 15 and October 10, Red's Meadow will pick up your packages at the Mammoth Lakes Post Office for $25. They visit the post office about four times per week. They will hold it at their general store for free for five days and for $1 per day thereafter. The store is open from 7 a.m. to 7 p.m. For more information and to download a resupply-request form, go to **www.redsmeadow.com.**

It is recommended that you mail your package first-class and that it not be more than 14 inches high, 14 inches wide, and 24 inches wide. Mail to:

[Your name]
c/o Red's Meadow Resort
P.O. Box 395
Mammoth Lakes, CA 93546

Vermilion Valley Resort

Vermilion Valley Resort receives more than 1,000 resupply packages per year for JMT and PCT thru-hikers. They visit the post office once or twice a week, so be sure your package arrives 10 to 14 days before you do. They charge $15 and the fee is collected upon pickup. Each package can weigh no more than 25 pounds, and will be held for 30 days. Unclaimed packages will be placed in the hikers box for other hikers in need of extra supplies. Packages can also be returned for a $10 charge, plus postage. For more information and updates, go to **www.edison lake.com.** Send your package via U.S. Mail (the preferred method) to:

[Your name]
[Your expected date of arrival]
Vermilion Valley Resort
P.O. Box 258
Lakeshore, CA 93634

Muir Trail Ranch

The Muir Trail Ranch receives about 400 food caches a year from June through September 15. Their very specific regulations on send-ing resupplies can be found at **www.muirtrailranch.com/resupply .html.** You need to package your food in a five-gallon plastic bucket with a snap lid to ensure airtightness and mouse-proofing. It costs

$45 to pick up each package, and the maximum weight is 25 pounds. Send your package so it will arrive at the post office two or three weeks ahead of your pickup date. Packages should be sent via Priority Mail with delivery confirmation to the following address:

[Your name]
[Your expected date of arrival and pickup]
[Your e-mail address]
c/o Muir Trail Ranch
P.O. Box 176
Lakeshore, CA 93634

Send check or money order payable to Muir Trail Ranch to:
MTR Resupply
P.O. Box 176
Lakeshore, CA 93634

Be sure that the name of the food-cache recipient accompanies the check. Packages will be held for 30 days.

Pack Outfitters

Another option for resupplying en route is to contact a pack station to bring in your food via horse, mule, or llama. This is an expensive option, with prices starting around $450 and going up steadily from there, depending on the number of animals needed and the duration of the trip. It can, however, provide you with a lot of options for layover days that a diminishing food supply can limit. In addition to resupply, these folks can also pack out your trash or carry your gear to your next campsite. All for a fee, of course. The Inyo National Forest has a list of pack stations at www.**fs.fed.us/r5/inyo/recreation/packstations.shtml.**

Two recommended establishments are **Rainbow Pack Outfitters** in Bishop, (760) 873-8877 or **www.rainbowpackoutfit.com,** and **Sequoia Kings Pack Trains** in Independence, (800) 962-0775 or (760) 387-2797, in business since 1872.

Yosemite
National Park

VERNAL AND NEVADA FALLS, HALF DOME, CATHEDRAL LAKES, LYELL CANYON

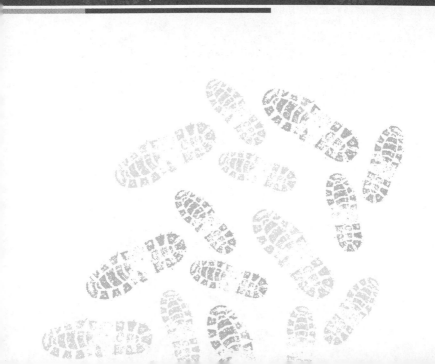

In the high altitude, you soar above the treeline with wide granite expanses and endless views. In lower elevations, relish the rich diversity of flora in sunny meadows and shady forest thickets. Throughout, find a range of lakes, streams, rivers, and distinct ecosystems

1 Vernal and Nevada Falls

SCENERY: ☆ ☆ ☆ ☆ ☆	DISTANCE: *8 miles*
TRAIL CONDITION: ☆ ☆ ☆ ☆	HIKING TIME: *4–6 hours*
CHILDREN: ☆ ☆ ☆	OUTSTANDING FEATURES: *Vernal Falls,*
DIFFICULTY: ☆ ☆ ☆	*Nevada Falls, Emerald Pool, Silver Apron, Clark*
SOLITUDE: ☆	*Point, sweeping views of the valley*

A Yosemite classic, this one has it all: rushing waterfalls, verdant canyons, slabs of imposing granite, shady conifers, and inspiring views of the valley below. Nevada Falls drops 594 feet, making it the longest single leap of the Merced River, while Vernal Falls completes the journey with a 317-foot drop.

The trail is no secret, but it's hard to blame the masses once you witness its dramatic charm. Start this walk early before it's overrun with valley-floor visitors, as well as to avoid midday heat in the summer. Beginning on the John Muir Trail (JMT), this is a balloon loop. Start by climbing to a scenic footbridge and a thunderous view of Vernal Falls. Next, continue up the Mist Trail to the top of Nevada Falls. To return, loop back, descending on the more gradual JMT to rejoin your route at the footbridge.

🥾 From the Happy Isles Shuttle Stop #16 (4,035 feet), walk along the road crossing the bridge over the Merced River and then turn right to follow the river south along the dusty, well-defined path. Follow the path as it ascends rather steeply along the river canyon and around Sierra Point, a rocky ledge on the southwest ridge of Grizzly Peak named after the Sierra Club. This is a fitting beginning to your hike, as John Muir was the first president elected to this conservation body in 1892. This is a crowded path, and you may be as amazed at the impressive variety of footwear—and the diverse smattering of accents from around the world—as you are with the granite boulders and distant waterfalls. As you ascend, pass through and above Happy Isles's woodland of conifers and live-oak trees.

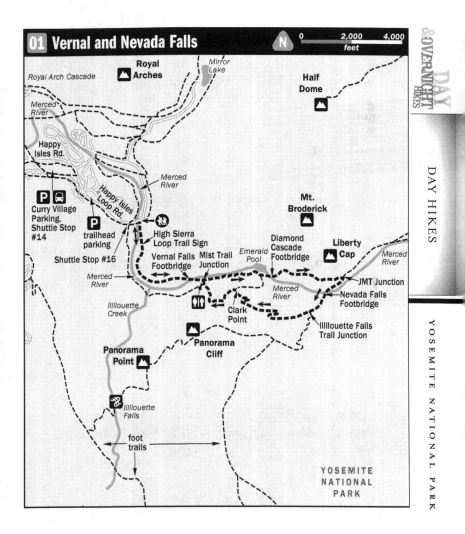

01 Vernal and Nevada Falls

N

0   2,000   4,000
feet

Royal Arch Cascade

Royal Arches

Mirror Lake

Merced River

Half Dome

Happy Isles Rd.

Merced River

Curry Village Parking, Shuttle Stop #14

Happy Isles Loop Rd.

trailhead parking

Shuttle Stop #16

High Sierra Loop Trail Sign

Vernal Falls Footbridge

Mist Trail Junction

Emerald Pool

Mt. Broderick

Diamond Cascade Footbridge

Liberty Cap

Merced River

Merced River

Merced River

JMT Junction

Nevada Falls Footbridge

Illilouette Creek

Clark Point

Illilouette Falls Trail Junction

Panorama Point

Panorama Cliff

Illilouette Falls

foot trails

YOSEMITE NATIONAL PARK

DAY & OVERNIGHT HIKES

DAY HIKES

YOSEMITE NATIONAL PARK

and above Happy Isles's woodland of conifers and live-oak trees. Within 0.75 miles, reach your first viewing point of Vernal Falls. Together, the two falls are known as the Grand Staircase, as the Merced River dramatically steps its way down to the valley.

Camera-toting tourists in flip-flops and bikini tops crowd a wooden footbridge located here (4,600 feet). Just across the bridge look for a drinking fountain, restrooms, and an army of brazen snack-marauding squirrels.

From this vantage point, you can see the final plunge of the Merced River, which collects winter runoff from Mount Lyell, Yosemite's highest peak at 13,114 feet. Witness the dramatic cascade year-round as water thunders down amid a frame of pine and cedar trees.

Shortly after leaving the footbridge, the trail reaches a junction. The Mist Trail continues on the left following the river along a rock-lined path through an area of lodgepole pines. The official John Muir Trail (JMT) turns to the right, taking a longer, more gradual climb before rejoining the shorter and steeper Mist Trail at the top of Nevada Falls.

Follow the Mist Trail eastward up-canyon with a spectacular view

ELEVATION PROFILE

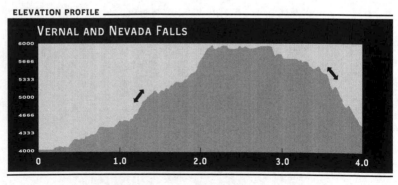

in the spring and early summer, living up to its name with watery mist drenching hikers as they make their way up hundreds of steep and sometimes slippery granite steps. Many hikers don raincoats for this section of the trail, but on a hot day the waterfall shower provides welcome relief. First reach the lower viewpoint of the falls, and then ascend the wet path upward, keeping your eyes peeled for rainbows in the spray.

At the top of Vernal Falls, a rail protects you from the sheer drop, hopefully keeping you from losing your camera, your lunch, or your life. Vernal means springtime, and the continual mist from the falls keeps the canyon lush and cool so that it's perennially springtime in this corridor. Just upriver of the overlook lie the stunning wading pools and cascading waters of the Emerald Pool and Silver Apron, the latter so named for its color as a continual sheet of water streams over flat slabs of smooth granite.

It's tempting to slide down the Silver Apron or swim here, but the current is incredibly strong and history shows repeatedly that disaster (as in death) is assured for those who attempt it. But a foot soak, head dunk, and scenic snack are all highly encouraged. You will find some composting restrooms upriver from the pools, just off the trail to the right.

Continue eastward and cross a wooden bridge over Diamond Cascade and then follow a relatively shaded gradual ascent, giving way to some exposed switchbacks in view of Nevada Falls. While the climb is steep up the rock walls, you have the prize in sight.

Reach a juncture with solar composting toilets and a series of trails leading to Half Dome, Cloud's Rest, and Tenaya Lake. For JMT thru-hikers, this is where the route continues toward Tuolumne.

Turn right to follow the JMT southwest back toward the valley and reach a wide wading area. Before crossing the bridge, you can access an observation platform footbridge that allows you a glimpse into the river's depths before it cascades violently over the edge. Many people miss this awesome overlook, which is worth a visit to really get a feel for the height. The iron-railed observation terrace is off a spur trail just north of the river. Nevada Falls flows through a narrow rock niche with tremendous force and then hits the wall, splitting into two different trajectories. After you've gotten your fill, rejoin the main trail and cross the wooden bridge (5,980 feet) to enjoy more dramatic views of the valley below.

Descend toward the valley and continue on the main path, ignoring cross trails to Illilouette Falls. Descend gradually, sometimes along a moist canyon wall that provides a bit of a light shower in the early season. This whole route was blasted from the canyon wall, and it's an impressive feat of modern engineering.

When you reach Clark Point (5,481 feet), take in the views of the falls and the towering monoliths of the Liberty Cap, the back of Half Dome, and Mount Broderick. Stay left to follow the JMT down a series of steep switchbacks dotted with gnarled oak trees amid the granite.

As you approach the river, keep right to stay on the foot trail as a stock trail descends to the left. As you near the river, turn left to follow the JMT back to the bridge, waterfalls, and bathrooms at the base of the falls, and return the way you came to the shuttle-bus stop.

PERMIT INFORMATION: *No permits necessary for day hikes*

DIRECTIONS: Yosemite can be entered via four main gateways: The BIG OAK FLAT ROAD ENTRANCE is on CA 120 West (Big Oak Flat Road) and is the closest western access to Tuolumne Meadows; the ARCH ROCK ENTRANCE on CA 140 (El Portal Road) is east of Merced and the safest bet in inclement weather, as it receives the least amount of snowfall; the SOUTH ENTRANCE is on CA 41 (Wawona Road), north of Fresno; and the weather-dependent TIOGA PASS ENTRANCE is on CA 120 East (Tioga Road) and is the closest eastern access to Tuolumne Meadows. Tioga Road is closed during the winter months due to snow, and sometimes doesn't open until June or July. While the first three entrances are generally open year-round, all roads are subject to closure; check with the park service by phone at (209) 372-0200 or visit www.nps.gov/yose/planyourvisit/ conditions.htm to determine current conditions.

The Happy Isles trailhead is in the southeastern part of Yosemite Valley, 1 mile past Curry Village. Year-round, day hikers are encouraged to leave their car in one of the day-use parking lots near Curry and Yosemite Villages and take the free shuttle bus to Shuttle Stop #16. There is a parking lot at Happy Isles, but it is often full in the summer months.

GPS coordinates	HAPPY ISLES
UTM zone (WGS84)	11S
Easting	0274558
Northing	4179230
Latitude	N 37°43'57.31"
Longitude	W 119°33'31.47"

2 Half Dome

SCENERY: ✪ ✪ ✪ ✪ ✪
TRAIL CONDITION: ✪ ✪ ✪ ✪
CHILDREN: ✪
DIFFICULTY: ✪ ✪ ✪ ✪ ✪
SOLITUDE: ✪
DISTANCE: 16.5 miles

HIKING TIME: 8–12 hours
OUTSTANDING FEATURES: Vernal and Nevada
falls, stupendous views of Yosemite Valley, steel cables
at top (late May–mid-October; do not attempt hike if
cables are down)

For many, Half Dome defines the Yosemite landscape; this stunning granite monolith appears in more scrapbooks worldwide than virtually any other peak. Reigning supremely over the valley floor at 8,842 feet, its looming form is unmistakable as it beckons hikers to a lofty 360-degree panorama. On the must-do list of nearly every California hiker, this is a challenging and long journey that features rushing rivers, turbulent waterfalls, and steep granite walls. The hike first ascends past Vernal and Nevada Falls to Little Yosemite Valley, plateaus briefly, then continues rising. The last 400 feet of the climb are the most memorable, as they include the infamous Half Dome cables that carry you up the final exposed pitch. But the real prize is the jaw-dropping view once you arrive, which should help you forget nearly all the pain of this 5,000-foot ascent.

For years, many thought it was impossible to reach the very top of Half Dome on foot. The 45-degree grade, combined with a slick and smooth rock face, made the feat seem unreachable. However, in 1875, George Anderson, a Scottish sailor lured to California with prospects of gold, was the first to prove naysayers wrong. Drilling holes into the granite, installing bolts, and using rope, Anderson attained his lofty goal, thus inspiring others to follow. John Muir was one of the first two dozen adventurers to follow his lead, and today nearly 500 people a day attempt the trek. In 1919, the Sierra Club erected the first set of cables for public use, and now the park maintains them each year. Do not attempt the climb if the cables are down, as it is quite dangerous. It is also important to note the weather before setting out; lightning hits the

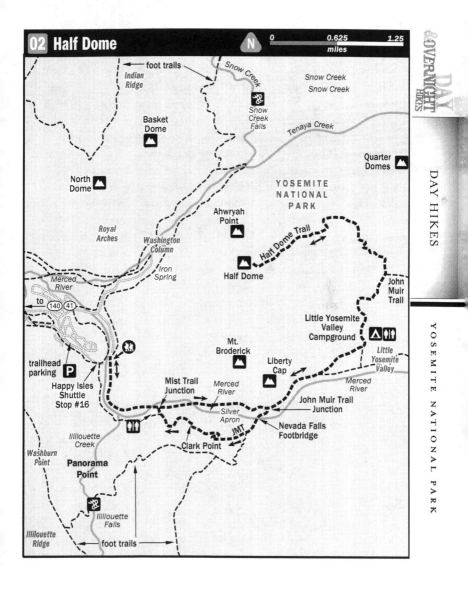

N

0   0.625   1.25
miles

foot trails

Snow Creek

Indian Ridge

Snow Creek
Snow Creek

Snow Creek Falls

Tenaya Creek

Basket Dome

Quarter Domes

North Dome

YOSEMITE NATIONAL PARK

Ahwryah Point

Half Dome Trail

Royal Arches

Washington Column

Half Dome

John Muir Trail

Iron Spring

Merced River

to 140 41

Little Yosemite Valley Campground

Little Yosemite Valley

trailhead parking P

Happy Isles Shuttle Stop #16

Mt. Broderick

Liberty Cap

Mist Trail Junction

Merced River

Merced River

John Muir Trail Junction

Silver Apron

Nevada Falls Footbridge

Illilouette Creek

JMT

Clark Point

Washburn Point

Panorama Point

Illilouette Falls

Illilouette Ridge

foot trails

33

dome every month of the year and the high, exposed ground leaves you nowhere to protect yourself.

If you are day hiking, be sure to bring plenty of water and a light, and layer your clothing. Temperatures can shift quickly in the mountains and it's best to be prepared. It's also best to get an early start before the sun, and the crowds, start hitting the mountain in full force.

From Happy Isles (4,035 feet), ascend steeply to the footbridge (4,600 feet). Shortly after the footbridge, there is a choice: The Mist Trail continues straight, hugging the river and ascending to Vernal Falls via a steep path that is often wet with waterfall spray, hence the name. This trail is more challenging on the knees with a short stretch bordered by a cable to help the climb. The other option is to veer right (east) and follow the John Muir Trail (JMT) on a more gradual climb through shaded switchbacks. The downside to taking this route is you miss the dramatic waterworks of the fall as seen from below. Our recommendation is to ascend via the Mist Trail and descend via the JMT, as both trails lead to the top of Nevada Falls' 600-foot drop. For a more detailed description of the hike up to Nevada Falls, see page 26 on this day hike. Combined, Vernal and Nevada falls make up the Grand Staircase, the name used to describe the tumultuous

ELEVATION PROFILE

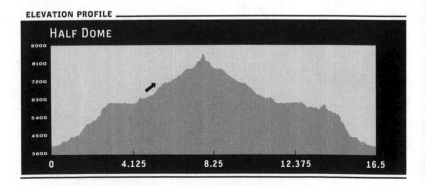

journey of the Merced River as it thunders its way down to the valley floor.

From Nevada Falls (5,980 feet), follow the JMT and come to a trail junction with solar toilets and many trails. Continue to climb gently on open rock to Little Yosemite Valley (6,140 feet), following the trail north-eastward. Shortly, the path turns dusty, and after about a mile the trail curves downhill to the first legal campground after leaving the valley floor. Stay left at the first junction, and soon reach the established campsites. If you need water, you can access the rushing Merced River just south of camp.

Rangers estimate that 20 percent of all backcountry campers in Yosemite pass through Little Yosemite Valley, so they appreciate your help in lessening the environmental impact by using the composting toilets and packing out all your trash. This overused area is rife with bears as well as aggressive squirrels and stellar blue jays, so keep an eye on your food. During the summer, a ranger is stationed just east of the campground on the other side of Sunshine Creek; a marked spur trail leads to the station off the JMT shortly after leaving the campground.

After leaving Little Yosemite Valley (6,140 feet), ascend moderately for 2.2 miles to the juncture with the Half Dome Trail (7,020 feet). Bypass the sign for the ranger station and continue climbing. The climb is moderately gradual until reaching the last half mile, which is a bit of a rock scramble up the northeast shoulder of the mountain. At times, the path is difficult to discern in the rock, but well-placed cairns keep you from losing your way. Basically as long as you keep going up, up, up, you're going the right way. Finally, reach the famed Half Dome cables. From late May to mid-October, two steel ropes are suspended at waist height from pipes set in the rock to assist the climb. There are also intermittent wooden cross boards that provide a much-needed ledge to rest upon while attempting the ascent up the 45-degree rock face. Do not attempt the climb when the cables aren't in place, as the rock is deceptively slick.

Choose a set of gloves from the pile at the base of the cables if you don't have your own, as serious cable burns are inevitable for the gloveless. For those with a fear of heights, the cable ascent can be a breathtaking experience, and we don't just mean the view. Take it slowly, as the cables are crowded in the peak season, and you may need to allow others to pass. The one consolation is that finally your arms get the workout instead of your legs. At the top, reach a wide expanse of nearly level rock stretching over five acres. For the brave of heart, belly up to the narrow overhanging northwest point, dubbed the Diving Board (8,836 feet), and stick your head over for an amazing view of the rock wall, maybe even coming face to face with a rock climber. Many rock climbers scale up the sheer face of the dome and "walk off the rock," meaning that they will hike down the same way you will.

Enjoy epic views in every direction: over the valley, back toward Cloud's Rest and the Sierra Crest. Tempting though it may be, camping is forbidden on the top of Half Dome. This is to protect the fragile ecosystem that is constantly being threatened by human waste, burned trees, and rocks being moved around for wind shelter. There is, however, a suitable (but dry) campground on the northeast shoulder about half a mile down on the trail from the summit.

Return the way you came. If you opt to descend via the gentler JMT from the top of Nevada Falls, follow the JMT over the foot-bridge crossing the Merced River and continue descending toward Clark Point. The observation point is named after Galen Clark, a homesteader who moved to Yosemite in 1853 after being diagnosed with consumption (tuberculosis) and was given a short amount of time to live. The magic of the mountains prevailed, Clark's lungs healed, and he went on to become the first to discover the Mariposa Grove of Giant Sequoia trees. A great advocate of early environmental-protection acts, Clark served as Guardian of Yosemite National Park for more than two decades.

In the early season, there is a nice cooling mist coming off the wall en route to this viewing point. From Clark's Point, enjoy a great backward panorama of the falls, as well as Liberty Cap and Grizzly Peak. Eventually rejoin the Mist Trail just above the footbridge at Vernal Falls. From here, follow the footbridge and return to the Happy Isles trailhead.

PERMIT INFORMATION: *No permits necessary for day hikes*

DIRECTIONS: Yosemite can be entered via four main gateways: The BIG OAK FLAT ROAD ENTRANCE is on CA 120 West (Big Oak Flat Road) and is the closest western access to Tuolumne Meadows; the ARCH ROCK ENTRANCE on CA 140 (El Portal Road) is east of Merced and the safest bet in inclement weather, as it receives the least amount of snowfall; the SOUTH ENTRANCE is on CA 41 (Wawona Road), north of Fresno; and the weather-dependent TIOGA PASS ENTRANCE is on CA 120 East (Tioga Road) and is the closest eastern access to Tuolumne Meadows. Tioga Road is closed during the winter months due to snow, and sometimes doesn't open until June or July. While the first three entrances are generally open year-round, all roads are subject to closure; check with the park service by phone at (209) 372-0200 or visit www.nps.gov/yose/planyourvisit/conditions.htm to determine current conditions.

The Happy Isles trailhead is in the southeastern part of Yosemite Valley, 1 mile past Curry Village. Year-round, day hikers are encouraged to leave their cars in one of the day-use parking lots near Curry and Yosemite Villages and take the free shuttle bus to Shuttle Stop #16. There is a parking lot at Happy Isles, but it is often full in the summer months.

GPS coordinates	HAPPY ISLES
UTM zone (WGS84)	11S
Easting	0274558
Northing	4179230
Latitude	N 37°43'57.31"
Longitude	W 119°33'31.47"

3 Cathedral Lakes

SCENERY: ✿ ✿ ✿ ✿	
TRAIL CONDITION: ✿ ✿ ✿ ✿	*include lower Cathedral Lake)*
CHILDREN: ✿ ✿ ✿	HIKING TIME: *4–5 hours*
DIFFICULTY: ✿ ✿ ✿	OUTSTANDING FEATURES: *Upper and lower*
SOLITUDE ✿	*Cathedral Lakes; stunning views of the Cathedral*
DISTANCE: *7 miles round-trip (8 miles if you*	*Range, including Cathedral Peak, as well as Echo and Tresidder peaks*

The Upper and Lower Cathedral Lakes are two alpine jewels glistening amidst the grandeur of their namesake mountain range. A 1,000-foot climb from Tuolumne Meadows, the gorgeous sister lakes sit regally in a classic glacial cirque. The hike begins in the shade of lodgepole pines and other neighboring conifers before opening up to more expansive views. The climb is never more than a moderate ascent, but it can still feel unrelenting on a hot day. Your reward is a cool dip in these picture-perfect lakes, two of the region's finest, with striking views of the surrounding peaks.

🐾 From the Cathedral Lakes trailhead (8,630 feet), follow the John Muir Trail (JMT) southwest away from Tioga Road. The trail designations can be tricky here, sometimes marked as the JMT, sometimes marked as Cathedral Lakes, and sometimes marked as Sunrise High Sierra Camp. Follow the trail up the initially dusty path away from the highway, and encounter a series of shaded switchbacks beneath fir and lodgepole pine trees that rise sharply for half a mile out of the meadow. Despite the initial shade, this is still best attempted before the midday heat.

As you gain altitude, the scenery changes from hemlock-strewn meadows and thatches of wood to broader expanses with views of granite giants. After a slight plateau, encounter a second push of moderate to steep grade. Cross Cathedral Creek and several springs while following the west flank of Cathedral Peak. The Cathedral Range separates the Tuolumne and Merced rivers. The range is

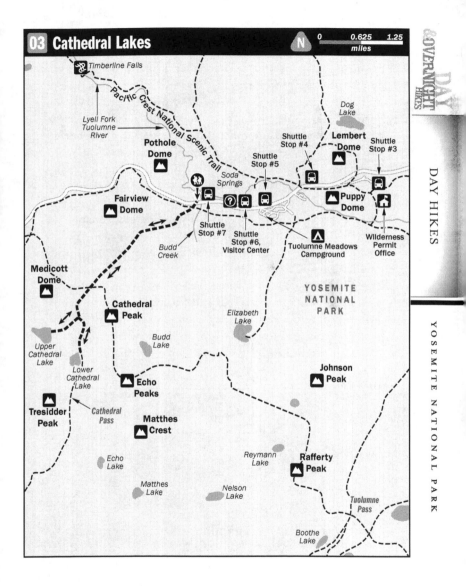

0   0.625   1.25
miles

N

Timberline Falls

Pacific Crest National Scenic Trail

Lyell Fork
Tuolumne
River

Dog
Lake

Pothole
Dome

Shuttle
Stop #4

Lembert
Dome

Shuttle
Stop #3

Shuttle
Stop #5

Soda
Springs

Fairview
Dome

Puppy
Dome

Shuttle
Stop #7

Budd
Creek

Shuttle
Stop #6,
Visitor Center

Tuolumne Meadows
Campground

Wilderness
Permit
Office

Medicott
Dome

Cathedral
Peak

Elizabeth
Lake

YOSEMITE
NATIONAL
PARK

Upper
Cathedral
Lake

Budd
Lake

Lower
Cathedral
Lake

Echo
Peaks

Johnson
Peak

Tresidder
Peak

Cathedral
Pass

Matthes
Crest

Echo
Lake

Reymann
Lake

Rafferty
Peak

Matthes
Lake

Nelson
Lake

Tuolumne
Pass

Boothe
Lake

DAY HIKES

YOSEMITE NATIONAL PARK

named for its celebrated peak, as glacial activity has given the mountain a distinctive double pinnacle outline reminiscent of a grand cathedral. As the horizontal view increases, look for the appropriately named Sawtooth Ridge with jagged spires and Matterhorn Peak.

Not surprisingly, this trail sees a lot of use, as it's a major thoroughfare for backpackers and day-trippers alike making their way into the backwoods via Tuolumne. Watch the trail to avoid horse manure, as this is the resupply route for pack trains traveling to Sunrise High Sierra Camp.

After 3 miles and just under 1,000 feet of climbing, the first juncture points to Upper Cathedral Lake to the right (west). A half-mile trail brings you through pine woods and hemlock shading to follow a rippling inlet stream that bounces along a meadow before reaching Lower Cathedral Lake (9,288 feet). Nestled snugly under the watchful eye of Cathedral Peak (10,840 feet), the lake is a photographer's dream. Lower Cathedral Lake tends to be the less crowded of the two, as many hikers and backpackers stay on the main John Muir Trail to Upper Cathedral Lake. But this spur trail is worth a detour to see this stunning subalpine beauty cradled in a granite bowl. If you brave an icy dip, there are plenty of broad rocky expanses

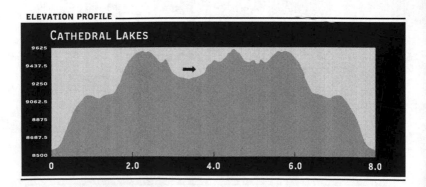

ELEVATION PROFILE

CATHEDRAL LAKES

where you can sit and warm yourself. After a wet winter season, be prepared for muddy and wet meadow walks en route to the lake in spring and early summer.

Return the way you came to the junction and continue up the trail another half mile toward Sunrise High Sierra Camp to reach Upper Cathedral Lake (9,585 feet). This sister lake is also ringed by granite, with a shallow sandy basin, and placid water reflecting the impressive form of Cathedral Peak. Look east to admire the dramatic neighboring pinnacles of Tresidder and Echo. The upper lake is said to have better fishing and is more popular with anglers.

Once again retracing your steps, it's a sandy 3.5 miles through wildflower-strewn meadows and shady switchbacks from Upper Cathedral Lake back to the trailhead.

PERMIT INFORMATION: *No permits necessary for day hikes*

DIRECTIONS: The Cathedral Lakes trailhead is in the Tuolumne Meadows area of Yosemite National Park off Tioga Road (CA 120 East). There is a parking area just south of CA 120, less than 2 miles west of the visitor center (Shuttle Stop #6). There is no formal lot here, just pullouts, so you may also opt to park at the visitor center and ride the bus to Shuttle Stop #7. This free park shuttle service runs from 7 a.m. to 6:30 p.m. along Tioga Road from Tuolumne Lodge to Olmsted Point from July 4 through Labor Day. You can also walk from the visitor center to the trailhead by heading east on the path found behind the visitor-center building until you reach the juncture with the Cathedral Lakes Trail (about 1 mile).

GPS coordinates	CATHEDRAL LAKES
UTM zone (WGS84)	11S
Easting	0290487
Northing	4194459
Latitude	N 37°52'24.75"
Longitude	W 119°22'55.46"

4 Lyell Canyon

SCENERY: ✪ ✪ ✪ ✪ ✪	SOLITUDE: ✪
TRAIL CONDITION: ✪ ✪ ✪ ✪ ✪	DISTANCE: 5–11 miles out and back
CHILDREN: ✪ ✪ ✪ ✪ ✪ (shorter distance	HIKING TIME: 3–5 hours
would be appropriate for children)	OUTSTANDING FEATURES: Stunning meadows,
DIFFICULTY: ✪ (mileage is flexible, as this is an	views of Kuna Crest, trout fishing
out-and-back hike)	

This out-and-back is an easy Sunday stroll and a perfect spot for beginning hikers, families, or anyone desiring a lazy amble in an amazingly beautiful setting. If we had to introduce skeptical friends to the joys of lacing up hiking boots, this would be the trail to pick. The trail is mostly flat, but boasts picture-perfect meadows framed by granite monoliths, as gorgeous as any you may find in at Yosemite National Park. Usually you have to really work to afford a view like this.

🚶🚶 This is an out-and-back walk, so you can truly make it as long as you'd like. The flattest section of the John Muir Trail, this path would be quick walking if it weren't for the fact that you undoubtedly will want to stop and take pictures, soak in the beauty, and perhaps take a dip in the river's cool waters.

From the Dog Lake Parking Lot (8,700 feet), cross the road and follow signs to the John Muir Trail. After half a mile, cross a bridge over the Dana Fork of the Tuolumne River. Shortly thereafter, a second bridge takes you over the Lyell Fork. About 1.5 easy miles from the trailhead, traverse rushing Rafferty Creek on a handsome footbridge (8,720 feet), and begin a beautiful stroll in and out of forest thickets and along the grassy expanse of Lyell Canyon. The area is named for Charles Lyell, a 19th-century lawyer turned geologist and good friend of Charles Darwin.

Up until the mid-1800s, with its outpouring of prospectors and explorers, Native Americans were the only people to enjoy the beauty of this region. Miwok and Mono Indians stopped in the area to trade

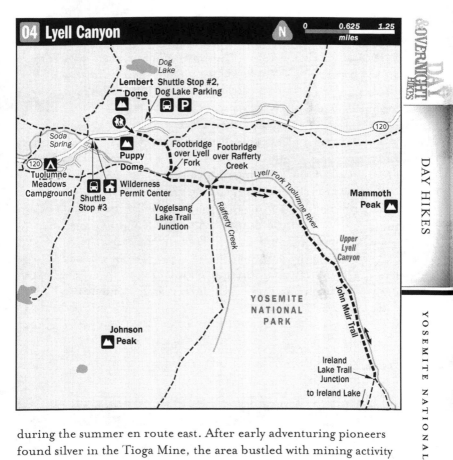

0   0.625   1.25
miles

Dog Lake

Lembert Dome

Shuttle Stop #2, Dog Lake Parking

Soda Spring

Puppy Dome

Footbridge over Lyell Fork

Footbridge over Rafferty Creek

Lyell Fork Tuolumne River

120

Tuolumne Meadows Campground

Shuttle Stop #3

Wilderness Permit Center

Vogelsang Lake Trail Junction

Rafferty Creek

Mammoth Peak

Upper Lyell Canyon

YOSEMITE NATIONAL PARK

Johnson Peak

John Muir Trail

Ireland Lake Trail Junction

to Ireland Lake

DAY HIKES

YOSEMITE NATIONAL PARK

during the summer en route east. After early adventuring pioneers found silver in the Tioga Mine, the area bustled with mining activity for several years. Today, the area still sees both a fair amount of trade and modern prospecting in the retail shops of the park.

The area is particularly lush in early season with an explosion of fiery wildflowers. Late April through mid-November, rainbow trout lure anglers to this stretch of Yosemite, while day hikers and picnickers hunker down by the river year-round.

The trail alternates between shady pockets of pine trees and open meadows, never rising more than 300 feet as it parallels the Lyell Fork of the Tuolumne River. The canyon is quite wide, so while there are imposing granite walls lining the meadow, it feels very open. Enjoy stunning views of the famed Unicorn Peak and farther along, Mount Lyell, the park's highest peak at 13,114 feet.

After crossing Rafferty Creek, reach your next trail junction in a little more than 4 miles at the turnoff (8,900 feet) for Ireland Lake and the designated return spot. Your walk brings you within feet of the shallow and gently flowing river that has been carving this valley for millions of years. Sometimes the water tumbles over giant rock slides, other times it meanders through grassland, and often it swirls into deep blue-green pools that invite a stop. Return the way you came, savoring views of Mammoth Peak and the Kuna Crest.

The trail's proximity to busy Tuolumne Meadows, as well as its level grade, nearly guarantees that you will have company in this part of the wilderness. The presence of hikers careless with their food, combined with shallow waters teeming with fish, also means that this is popular bear and deer country. Be sure to keep your food secure at all times.

PERMIT INFORMATION: *No permits necessary for day hikes*

ELEVATION PROFILE

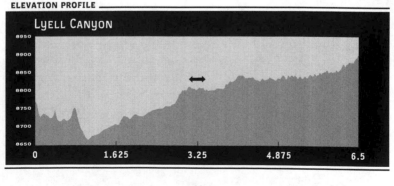

DIRECTIONS: The Lyell Canyon trailhead is in the Tuolumne Meadows area of Yosemite National Park off Tioga Road (CA 120). For parking, follow signs to the Tuolumne Lodge and Wilderness Permit office. There is a parking lot on the left signposted for Dog Lake and the John Muir Trail, or you may find additional parking in the Wilderness Permit lot and then follow the signs to the John Muir Trail. The park runs a free shuttle-bus service from 7 a.m. to 6:30 p.m. along Tioga Road from Tuolumne Lodge to Olmsted Point from July 4 through Labor Day; the Lyell Canyon trailhead can be found at Shuttle Stop #2. Additionally, YARTS bus service offers a shuttle from Tuolumne Meadows Visitor Center back to the Yosemite Village Visitor Center at 9:10 a.m. during the summer months. Rates are $15 one-way. Contact YARTS by phone at (888) 89-YARTS or visit www.yarts.com) for current rates and schedules.

GPS coordinates	Lyell Canyon
UTM zone (WGS84)	11S
Easting	0294479
Northing	4194386
Latitude	N 37°52'39.09"
Longitude	W 119°20'32.58"

Devils Postpile
National Monument
DEVILS POSTPILE AND
RAINBOW FALLS

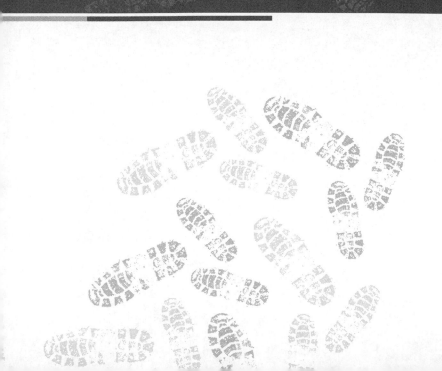

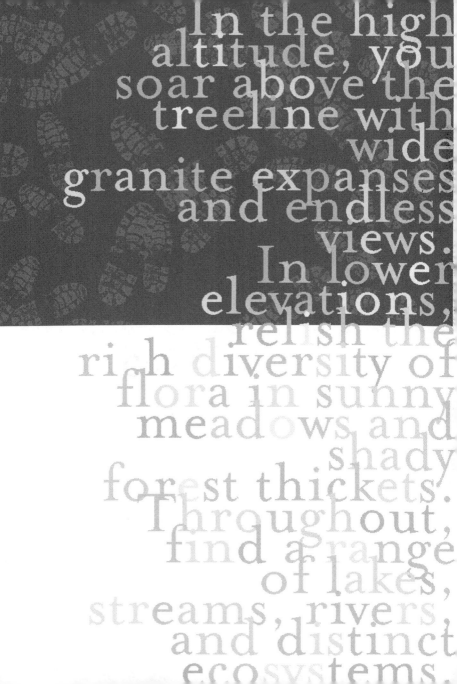

In the high altitude, you soar above the treeline with wide granite expanses and endless views. In lower elevations, relish the rich diversity of flora in sunny meadows and shady forest thickets. Throughout, find a range of lakes, streams, rivers, and distinct ecosystems

5 Devils Postpile **and Rainbow Falls**

SCENERY: ✿ ✿ ✿	DISTANCE: 6 miles
TRAIL CONDITION: ✿ ✿ ✿ ✿	HIKING TIME: 3–4 hours
CHILDREN: ✿ ✿ ✿ ✿	OUTSTANDING FEATURES: Basaltic-rock
DIFFICULTY: ✿	formations of Devils Postpile, Upper and Lower
SOLITUDE: ✿	Rainbow Falls, abundant bird life

The Devils Postpile is one of the most impressive examples of columnar basalt in the world. In layman's terms, this unique geologic formation is created by volcanic lava flow that cooled, shrunk, and fractured uniformly. The closest rival of any magnitude is the Giants Causeway in Northern Ireland, and after witnessing the mathematical precision of Devils Postpile hexagonal columns you'll understand why these natural displays are given such otherworldly names. This easy day hike also brings you past upper and lower Rainbow Falls, the former renowned for its 101-foot drop of water and the frequent rainbows that appear in its misty spray. Additionally, you will experience a burn-scarred area rich with bird life and regrowth.

🚶 The trail begins at the Rainbow Falls Trailhead, Shuttle Stop #9 (7,600 feet). Begin by descending dusty pumice through the Rainbow Fire area, cross a footbridge, and continue walking downhill. The easy accessibility, short distance, and gentle terrain make this a popular hike for kids and day-trippers. While the immediate landscape is scorched, the views of the mountains are expansive and broad. Of the trees that do remain, many are lodgepole pines, so named by Lewis and Clark when they saw them being used by Native Americans in their teepee construction.

In August 1992, fire swept through this region, destroying more than 8,000 acres. Dubbed the Rainbow Fire, due to its proximity to the waterfalls, the blaze resulted from a lightning strike and the ensuing winds that stirred the embers days later. Once roaring, it took

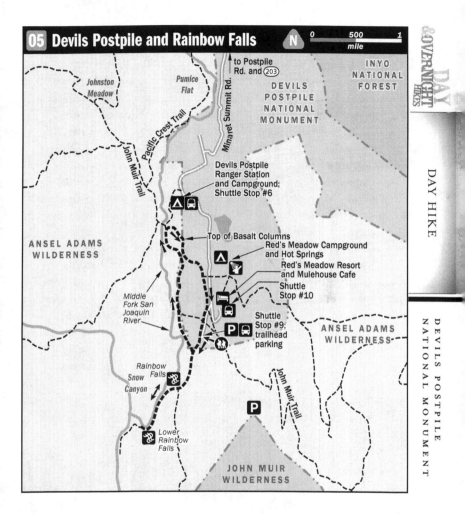

05 Devils Postpile and Rainbow Falls

N

0   500   1
mile

to Postpile
Rd. and (203)

INYO
NATIONAL
FOREST

Johnston
Meadow

Pumice
Flat

DEVILS
POSTPILE
NATIONAL
MONUMENT

Devils Postpile
Ranger Station
and Campground;
Shuttle Stop #6

Top of Basalt Columns

Red's Meadow Campground
and Hot Springs

Red's Meadow Resort
and Mulehouse Cafe

Shuttle
Stop #10

Shuttle
Stop #9;
trailhead
parking

ANSEL ADAMS
WILDERNESS

Middle
Fork San
Joaquin
River

ANSEL ADAMS
WILDERNESS

John Muir Trail

Rainbow
Falls

Snow
Canyon

Lower
Rainbow
Falls

P

JOHN MUIR
WILDERNESS

nearly two months before the last hot spots were extinguished. The ground cover served as fuel while the winds spread the damage, and scores of hikers were evacuated. However, it's not all dire news. Forest fires are natural occurrences, and the tree snags that remain standing serve as an important and desirable habitat for bird species. Additionally, the opened forest canopy means that more sunlight reaches the ground, allowing for greater diversity of plant life.

Follow the trail as it parallels a fork of the San Joaquin River, vibrant lupine lining the banks, and continue descending to Rainbow Falls (7,400 feet), a dramatic sheet of water cascading down 101 feet. There is an overlook from which to admire this incredible example of water's force, and the brilliant display of rainbows in the mist aptly gives meaning to the falls' name.

It's possible to walk down to the waterfall's base, where many enjoy wading and fishing in the cool jetty of water. Or continue along the trail to another stone observation platform. The waterfall's dramatic event is owed to two different types of volcanic rocks. The top layer of stone is a more robust, erosion-resistant rock, while the bottom layer is softer and more susceptible to the continuing cascade of water. This undercutting process gradually creates an alcove

ELEVATION PROFILE

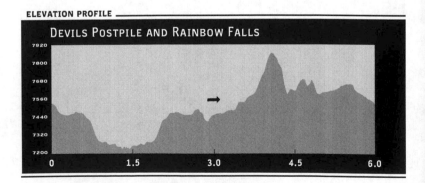

DEVILS POSTPILE AND RAINBOW FALLS

beneath the stronger rock layer that eventually caves in, hence the debris at the bottom of the falls.

To access the lower falls, turn left at your first opportunity to continue heading southwest along the trail. Most visitors ignore this trail, but, while less dramatic, Lower Rainbow Falls (7,200 feet) offers a bit more solitude and is the perfect spot for dipping your feet in the rushing river while picnicking. There is also a small swimming hole just below the fall for those willing to brave a dip. It's a serene landscape as granite boulders tumble into the river, and cottonwoods, willows, and alders sway in the breeze. Descending through a pine forest, there are many tree snags attracting roosting birds, while closer to the river, cow parsnip and redbud are scattered within the grasses.

Return the way you came, climbing gently through conifers on a pumice path. Numerous side trails lead to Red's Meadow, and the return walk provides clear views of Mammoth Mountain's bald backside.

Follow signs to Devils Postpile and continue to climb gently along the dusty trail. Interestingly, the 800 acres of Devils Postpile National Monument were originally considered a part of Yosemite National Park in 1890. However, aggressive efforts made by mining interests reversed this decision, and in 1905, Congress removed the site from the National Park. Five years later, the Forest Service was approached by those who wanted to create a rock dam on the San Joaquin River to power the electricity of their mining operations—a move that would require the dynamiting of Devils Postpile. Luckily, the Sierra Club, along with University of California professor Joseph LeConte, responded with their own lobbying efforts to President Taft, and the area was saved. Christened a National Monument in 1911, the area once again enjoys federal protection.

At the juncture with the base of Devils Postpile (7,560 feet), turn right to follow a sign to the top of the columns and begin a short series of switchbacks to see the basaltic rock formations from above. Like a granite garden of paving stones, it's hard to believe that the uniformly hexagonal stones were not cut by hand. The columns were exposed when a glacier traveled down the Middle Fork of the San Joaquin River some 10,000 to 20,000 years ago, carving away a side of the postpile and exposing the sheer wall of columns that we see today. The parallel grooves on the top of the stones are scrapes from rocks trapped in the slow-moving glacier. Looking across the river, there are views of lush Johnston Meadow.

Loop around, descending, and come to another junction. The north trail to the right leads to the Devils Postpile Ranger Station, Campground, and Shuttle Stop #6. A free shuttle from here leads back to the trailhead (Shuttle Stop #9) for any weary walkers. Otherwise, turn left and return toward the rock formations, passing in front of the basalt columns. The trail begins a short, moderate ascent before reaching a juncture with a trail toward Red's Meadow or Rainbow Falls. Follow the signs back to Red's Meadow Resort to return to the starting trailhead.

PERMIT INFORMATION: *No permits necessary for day hikes*

DIRECTIONS: Devils Postpile National Monument can be reached from Mammoth Lakes. From the Mammoth Ranger Station and Visitor Center (on CA 203, 3 miles west of US 395), head west on Main Street for 1.5 miles and turn right to continue on CA 203 (Minaret Road), climbing nearly 5 miles to Mammoth Mountain Inn.

During the summer months, you cannot access Devils Postpile National Monument via car from 7 a.m. to 7:30 p.m. unless you have campground or resort reservations, a handicap placard, or a special permit. Wilderness permits do not allow you vehicular access. Mandatory shuttles operate from the parking area in front of Mammoth Mountain Inn, beginning at 7:15 a.m. Tickets can be purchased at the Gondola Building in the Main Lodge; the 45-minute shuttle to the Devils Postpile area is free for children under age 3, $4 for children ages 3 to 15, and $7 for adults. Shuttle service within the national-monument area between campgrounds and trailheads is free, and the Rainbow Falls Trailhead is Shuttle Stop #9. For more information, contact the Mammoth Ranger Station and Visitor Center at (760) 924-5500 or visit the city's regional-transit site at www.ci.mammoth-lakes.ca.us/transit/regional_transit.htm.

If you have reservations or are traveling in the off-season (October to early June), continue driving up the hill to the Minaret Summit Entrance Station (9,175 feet) and follow the steep, narrow road the remaining 7 miles to the Devils Postpile Monument Area, Red's Meadow, trailheads, and campgrounds. The Rainbow Falls Trailhead is the last turnoff on your right as you head south toward Red's Meadow Resort.

GPS coordinates	Rainbow Falls
UTM (WGS84) zone	11S
Easting	0316528
Northing	4164310
Latitude	N 37°36'29.20"
Longitude	W 119°04'42.56"

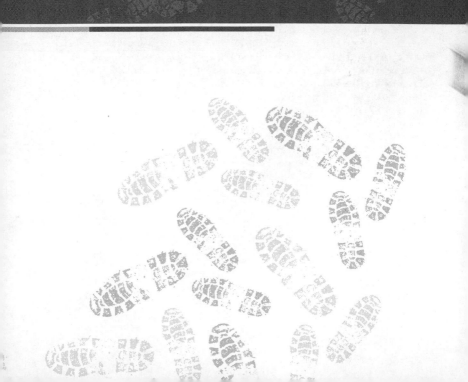

Sequoia
National Park
MOUNT WHITNEY

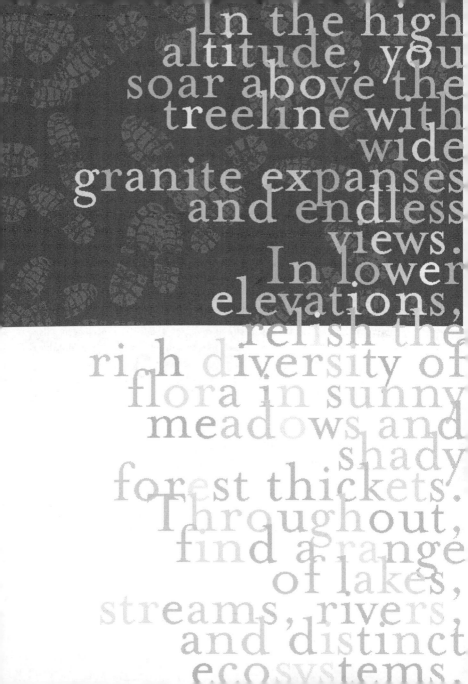

In the high altitude, you soar above the treeline with wide granite expanses and endless views. In lower elevations, relish the rich diversity of flora in sunny meadows and shady forest thickets. Throughout, find a range of lakes, streams, rivers and distinct ecosystems

6 Mount Whitney

SCENERY: ✿ ✿ ✿ ✿ ✿	DISTANCE: *22 miles*
TRAIL CONDITION: ✿ ✿ ✿ ✿	HIKING TIME: *1–3 days*
CHILDREN: ✿	OUTSTANDING FEATURES: *Mirror Lake,*
DIFFICULTY: ✿ ✿ ✿ ✿ ✿	*Trail Crest, Mount Whitney*
SOLITUDE: ✿	

*Anna Mills, the first woman to climb Mount Whitney in 1878, wrote of her journey,
"I can candidly say that I have never seen, nor do I expect to see, a picture so varied,
so sublime, so awe-inspiring, as that seen from the summit of Mount Whitney."*
(Mount Whitney Club Journal, 1902). *Indeed, Mount Whitney is a perch that
inspires the use of superlatives. Less intimidating than most peaks, Mount Whitney
welcomes hikers to her gently sloped top with a winding path that requires no technical
experience. As 14,000-foot mountains go, Mount Whitney is a relatively easy one to
climb. But relative is the key word. Hiking to the top of the highest peak in the lower
48 states (second in the continental United States only to Alaska's Mount McKinley),
is still a feat to be admired. Thin air, winding switchbacks, endless sun, and wind
exposure can all take their toll, and this is not a task to be taken lightly. Preparation—
both mental and physical—is the key to success. From trailhead to summit requires
more than 6,000 feet of elevation gain over 11 miles. The fittest of trail runners
accomplish the feat in less than three hours. But your average hiker will need any-
where from 12 to 16 hours to make the journey.*

🚶🚶 Begin at Whitney Portal (8,365 feet), stocking up on snacks
and water before departing. We've listed this as a day hike, as most
attempt to summit Whitney in this fashion, but truthfully we advise
an overnight stay en route to acclimate to the altitude and to be healthy
enough to enjoy the unparalleled view from the top. Day hikers should
start before sunrise to maximize daylight for the journey. Layered
clothing, plenty of water and food, sunscreen, and a light source are
all requirements. After a little more than a half mile of walking,

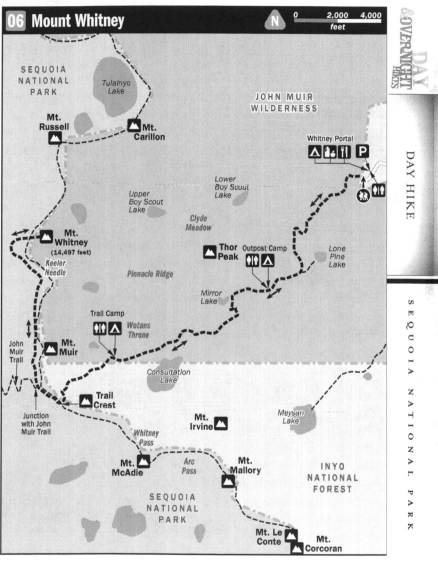

enter John Muir Wilderness and begin a series of steep open switch-backs through manzanita and stands of mountain mahogany and pine. Rock-hop across Lone Pine Creek and follow the creek on its southern bank. Ignore the unmarked spur trail leading to the right unless you plan on scaling the eastern face of Mount Whitney with mountaineering gear. There is a signed junction to Lone Pine Lake a little more than 2.5 miles from the trailhead. This is the closest camping to the trailhead, and it's a lovely spot with fewer crowds than subsequent campgrounds. To sleep here, simply follow the path less than a half mile to tent sites by the lake.

From the main trail, continue west up sandy sage-scented switchbacks and along a ridge, before descending slightly into the flower-strewn meadow of Bighorn Park. Traverse the south side of the meadow to cross Lone Pine Creek again and reach Outpost Camp (10,367 feet) nearly 4 miles from the trailhead at Whitney Portal. Crowded tent sites and solar toilets provide a halfway home for many hikers. If you camp here, you can leave your heavy gear at base camp to lighten your load up the mountain. In recent years, the toilets have not been able to keep up with the number of hikers, and they are often full toward the end of the season. In 2006, more than

ELEVATION PROFILE

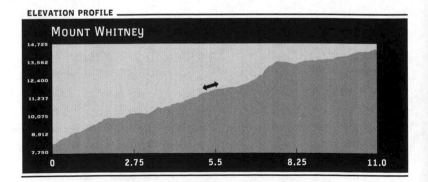

30,000 people camped in the Whitney Zone alone. As a result, the forest service is asking all backpackers to pick up "pack-it-out" kits and pack out *all* their trash. These glamorous "wag bags" come with toilet paper, hand sanitizer, and deodorant gel. There are disposal bins at Whitney Portal upon return to the trailhead. While it's less than spectacular to have to carry your wag bag with you, you can rest easy in the knowledge that you're aiding environmental progress.

Continue climbing up switchbacks to cross the outlet of Mirror Lake (10,640 feet), a gorgeous spot for a rest by its reflective waters. Camping is prohibited. Continue climbing up, through stunted white-bark pines, to rise above the treeline and arrive at Trailside Meadow. Continue rising up the granite landscape. Enjoy views of Consultation Lake to the south. Ascend poured concrete stairs to Trail Camp (12,000 feet). Listen for the high-pitched call of pikas— small, tailless, rabbitlike animals with laid-back ears—that frequent the area.

Trail Camp, the last legal camping area with water, lies close to 2,500 feet, and more than 4 miles below, Whitney. It is not without charm and enjoys lovely sunsets over a small tarn; however, it's a far cry from remote backcountry wilderness. Often overcrowded with inexperienced backpackers, it can feel a bit like a garbage dump at times. There are solar toilets on the southern side of camp, but these can sometimes be full. Whether camping or not, it is advised to pump water at this tarn, as this is the last water source before the summit.

Begin the famed 96 switchbacks up a relentless 2.3 miles to Trail Crest (13,650 feet) and the boundary for Sequoia National Park. The ascent begins with a tight set of steep switchbacks dynamited into the eastern side of the mountain. About halfway up, there are cables to assist hikers over ice when necessary. From the crest, admire views west to Sawtooth Peak and the Hitchcock Lakes and east to Owens Valley. Continuing from Trail Crest, enter Sequoia National Park leaving John Muir Wilderness. Enjoy a brief half-mile descent to Trail Junction (13,484 feet), where the John Muir Trail joins from the west to summit Mount Whitney. Turn right to begin the final 1.9-mile push to the summit over a stony ridge with the occasional peekaboo view of Owens Valley below to the east. While it's just shy of 2 miles to the top, with only about 1,000 feet of climbing at a moderate to gentle grade, the thin air makes the journey quite taxing.

Begin walking the rocky ridgeline, enjoying westward views to Mounts Hale and Young and beyond, and the pointed spire of Mount Muir to the east. Rocky spires and narrow ledges provide endless photo opportunities. The climb can be a bit vertigo-inducing for some, so take it easy and admire the jagged landscape of stony outcroppings, narrow windows with views to Owens Valley and asymmetrical rocks balanced in a seemingly precarious fashion on impossible ledges.

Round the corner around Keeler Needle, and begin the final ascent to the top of Mount Whitney (14,497 feet). Approaching the summit's broad plateau, it can be easy to lose the trail among the rocks. Watch for cairns until the tin-roofed shelter at the top comes into view. The shelter is a welcome spot during high winds, but do not seek protection here during a storm, as the tin roof is a lightning conductor. Hikers have died here in the past.

In the native tongue of the Owens Valley Paiute Indians, Mount Whitney was known as the "very old man." The Native Americans believed that the spirit of destiny lived in the mountain and observed their behavior from this grand perch. And indeed, the mountain has beckoned men and women to its airy crown for hundreds of years. Although it is sometimes disputed, it is generally acknowledged that the first people to ascend Mount Whitney were three fishing buddies from Lone Pine, in 1873: Charles Begole, Albert Johnson, and Johnny Lucas. They first climbed Mount Langley, realized it wasn't the tallest, and set a course for Whitney, dubbing it Fisherman's Peak. But the mountain had already been christened Mount Whitney in 1864 to honor Josiah Whitney, founder of the California Geological Survey and the author of a travel guide on Yosemite published in 1869. Despite the usual first-ascent naming rights, Mount Whitney remained the official moniker to honor this influential conservationist.

There's a palpable sense of victorious accomplishment in the air from all who reach the summit. Sign the guest book, housed in a steel box outside the shelter, that reveals the broad spectrum of ages and ethnicities that travel to Whitney's top. There is also a USGS survey marker to the east of the shelter among the big boulders. Older guidebooks mention a pit toilet at the top of the summit, but human waste has become a problem, and this is no longer encouraged.

Flanked by neighboring 14,000 footers Mounts Muir and Russell, Mount Whitney is a benign ruler towering above the Owens Valley. To the east, enjoy views of the Inyo Mountains and the Alabama Hills. To the south, Mount Hitchcock and Mount Langley greet the eye. To the west, admire the Sawtooth Peak, Kaweah Peaks, and the Great Western Divide. To the north lie Junction Peak, Mount Tyndall, and Mount Williamson, which just barely missed being the highest peak in the lower 48.

Keep your celebration in check, however, because it's important to conserve some energy for the descent. It's recommended that you leave the summit no later than 3 p.m., as it's still a more than 6,000-foot descent, and you want to have your wits (and humor) still about you when you return to civilization at Whitney Portal. Public restrooms are directly across from the trailhead, while food, showers (fee), a pay phone, and the general store are found to the right. The burger and fries combination is a treat! The general store is open daily (May and October, 9 a.m. to 6 p.m.; June and September, 8 a.m. to 8 p.m.; July and August, 7 a.m. to 9 p.m.).

Inspired? Next time you could choose to participate in the Bad-water Ultramarathon race, a 135-mile nonstop journey every July from Death Valley, the lowest elevation in the Western Hemisphere at

DAY HIKE

SEQUOIA NATIONAL PARK

280 feet below sea level, to the top of Mount Whitney. Those who manage to complete the journey in less than 48 hours are awarded a sought-after belt buckle celebrating their accomplishments.

PERMIT INFORMATION: *Because of the high demand to climb Mount Whitney, a quota system is in place from May 1 to November 1 for the Whitney Zone (the area stretching from Lone Pine Lake to Crabtree Meadow). During this time, 60 backpackers and 100 day hikers are allowed on the trail each day, and hikers must apply for a $15-per-person permit by entering the Mount Whitney Lottery. Lottery applications are accepted only during the month of February and must be mailed to the Wilderness Permit Office (351 Pacu Lane, Suite 200, Bishop, CA 93514). Applications must be postmarked in February and cannot be faxed to be eligible. Applications are available online at* **www.fs.fed.us/r5/inyo/recreation/wild/whitneylottery.shtml.** *To request that an application form be sent to you by mail or fax, call the Wilderness Permit Office at (760) 873-2483. The office is open from 8 a.m. to 4:30 p.m. daily from June 1 to October 1, and Monday through Friday during the rest of the year. You will be notified of your lottery status in April; rejected applications will be returned by mail.*

If you don't win the lottery, all hope is not lost. You can contact the Wilderness Permit Office two days before your trip to see if there is any remaining quota space. Walk-in permits are also available in the event of cancellations or no-shows. These permits are made available at 11 a.m. the day before the entry date at the Eastern Sierra InterAgency Visitor Center (junction of US 395 and CA 136), 2 miles south of Lone Pine. The center is open 8 a.m. to 6 p.m. Monday through Friday and can be reached by phone at (760) 876-6200. From November 2 to April 30, crowds are not a problem and permits may be self-issued at the visitor center.

DIRECTIONS: Whitney Portal lies 13 miles west of Lone Pine, off US 395, at the end of Whitney Portal Road. There is no public transit to the portal itself, but every car that leaves the parking lot goes through Lone Pine, so it's fairly easy to hitch a ride.

You can take public transit as far as Lone Pine via Inyo Mono Transit's CREST bus. It travels from Lone Pine south 1.5 hours to Ridgecrest and north to Bishop (1 hour) or Mammoth Lakes (2 hours). From Bishop, it's possible to transfer to another bus farther north to Reno. Rates and routes are subject to frequent change; call ahead for information and reservations at (760) 872-1901 or (800) 922-1930. More information can be found on the Web at www.countyofinyo.org/transit/CRESTpage.htm.

GPS coordinate	Whitney Portal
UTM zone (WGS84)	11S
Easting	0388918
Northing	4049743
Latitude	N 36°35'12.14"
Longitude	W 118°14'30.21"

Yosemite National Park and Ansel Adams Wilderness

**YOSEMITE VALLEY,
TUOLUMNE MEADOWS,
RED'S MEADOW**

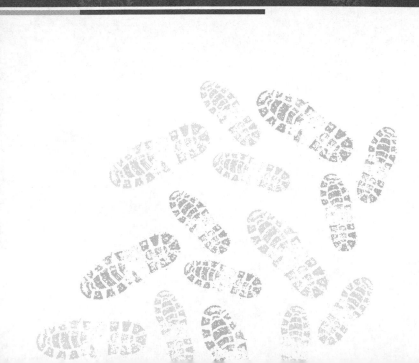

In the high altitude, you soar above the treeline with wide granite expanses and endless views. In lower elevations, relish the rich diversity of flora in sunny meadows and shady forest thickets. Throughout, find a range of lakes, streams, rivers, and distinct ecosystems

SCENERY: ☆ ☆ ☆ ☆	DISTANCE: *28 miles*
TRAIL CONDITION: ☆ ☆ ☆ ☆	HIKING TIME: *2–3 days*
CHILDREN: ☆ ☆ *(for kids used to*	OUTSTANDING FEATURES: *Nevada Falls,*
backcountry camping)	*an optional side visit to Half Dome, Little*
DIFFICULTY: ☆ ☆ ☆ ☆	*Yosemite Valley, Long Meadow, Cathedral Pass,*
SOLITUDE: ☆	*Cathedral Lakes*

The difficult first section of the John Muir Trail (JMT) climbs close to 6,000 feet over 28 miles as you make your way from the valley floor to Tuolumne Meadows. However this leg is also full of all the jaw-dropping scenery, sheer cliffs, and alpine meadows that make Yosemite a park virtually unparalleled in beauty. This is one of the least secluded stretches along the JMT, as many day- and weekend-trippers enter the park from both the start and end trailheads. However, even a crowd can't keep you from enjoying the incredible granite splendor of Yosemite.

Begin by climbing 2,000 feet to the top of the thundering Nevada Falls. From there, continue on a sandy plateau along the Merced River to Little Yosemite Valley, the first legal camping area. Continue ascending and begin following Sunrise Creek. Once you pass the spur trails for Half Dome and Cloud's Rest, the crowds thin, allowing pleasantly lonely up-river walks. The next big ascent leads to a bench above graceful Long Meadow. The final climb takes you up to Cathedral Pass, which is followed by a long descent through meadows and past subalpine lakes, to the visitor center in Tuolumne Meadow.

🚶🚶 From the Happy Isles Shuttle Stop #16 (4,035 feet), walk along the road crossing the bridge over the Merced River and then turn right to follow the river south along the dusty, well-defined path. Within a quarter mile, pass a sign for the High Sierra Loop that charts a journey that includes the mileage of the entire John Muir Trail to Mount Whitney (211 miles!). Follow the path as it ascends rather steeply along the river canyon and around Sierra Point, a rocky ledge

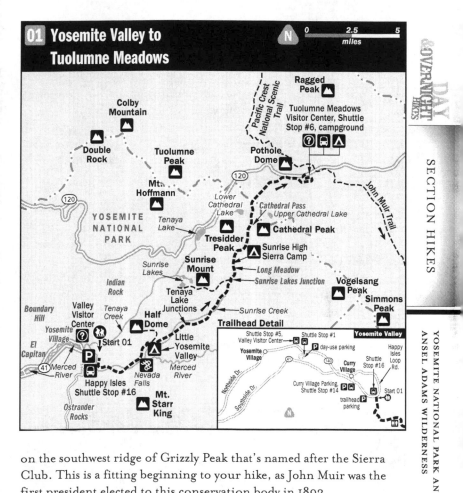

01 Yosemite Valley to Tuolumne Meadows

N   0   2.5   5
miles

Ragged Peak

Tuolumne Meadows Visitor Center, Shuttle Stop #6, campground

Colby Mountain

Double Rock

Tuolumne Peak

Pothole Dome

120

Mt. Hoffmann

Lower Cathedral Lake

Cathedral Pass
Upper Cathedral Lake

John Muir Trail

Pacific Crest National Scenic Trail

YOSEMITE NATIONAL PARK

120

Tenaya Lake

Cathedral Peak

Tresidder Peak

Sunrise High Sierra Camp

Sunrise Mount

Long Meadow

Sunrise Lakes Junction

Vogelsang Peak

Sunrise Lakes

Indian Rock

Tenaya Lake Junctions

Simmons Peak

Sunrise Creek

Boundary Hill

Valley Visitor Center

Tenaya Creek

Half Dome

Trailhead Detail

Shuttle Stop #5, Valley Visitor Center

Shuttle Stop #1

Yosemite Valley

Yosemite Village

El Capitan

41

Merced River

Start 01

Little Yosemite Valley

Nevada Falls

Merced River

Yosemite Village

day-use parking

41

140

Curry Village

Happy Isles Loop Rd.

Shuttle Stop #16

Northside Dr.

Southside Dr.

Curry Village Parking, Shuttle Stop #14

Shuttle Stop #16

Start 01

trailhead parking

Happy Isles Shuttle Stop #16

Mt. Starr King

Ostrander Rocks

on the southwest ridge of Grizzly Peak that's named after the Sierra Club. This is a fitting beginning to your hike, as John Muir was the first president elected to this conservation body in 1892.

Within less than a mile, reach a wooden footbridge (4,600 feet) and a view of the base of Vernal Falls. Together, Vernal and Nevada Falls are known as the Grand Staircase, as the Merced River dramatically steps its way down to the valley.

Just across the bridge is a drinking fountain with the last potable water before Tuolumne, restrooms, and a literal army of brazen snack-marauding squirrels. Shortly after leaving the footbridge, watch for a junction. The Mist Trail continues on the left, following the river steeply up wet and sometimes slippery granite steps in the spray of Vernal Falls. We recommend turning right to follow the John Muir Trail (JMT) up a longer, more gradual climb suitable for back-packers. This route follows the canyon's south wall under the shade of conifers and bigleaf maples before rejoining the shorter and steeper Mist Trail at the top of Nevada Falls.

Shortly after the switchbacks begin, a pack trail enters from the right; ignore the pack trail and continue ascending through Douglas fir and oak trees. After 2 miles, reach Clark Point (5,481 feet), so named for Galen Clark, one of the first guardians of Yosemite National Park and the first to discover the Mariposa Grove of Giant Sequoia near Wawona. From here, soak in views of the falls, Mount Broderick, and the Liberty Cap. Continuing up, the trail begins to hug the moist canyon wall, sometimes literally dripping with water in the spring and early summer. The path flattens and then dips a bit before emerging at a footbridge (5,980 feet) atop the falls. Look for

ELEVATION PROFILE

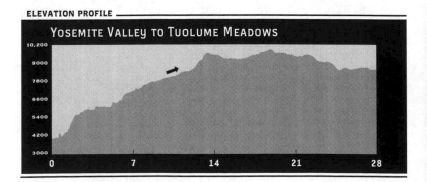

the iron-railed observation terrace located off of a spur trail just north of the river. Many people miss the awesome overlook, which is worth a visit to really get a feel for the height.

Once you've had a chance to soak your feet and battle the squirrels and stellar blue jays who want your peanuts, continue heading northeast on the rock-lined path. Within ten minutes, you'll pass a junction with the Mist Trail as well as some composting toilets.

Continue to climb gently northeastward to Little Yosemite Valley (6,140 feet). Shortly, the path turns dusty, and after about a mile the trail curves downhill toward the campground. At a Y juncture, notice that you can continue either way to the campsites; the split trail rejoins near the composting toilets of the site. The path that heads right is considered the official JMT route and parallels the Merced River. The path that heads left is the more direct route for hikers continuing to Half Dome. Either trail leads to the composting toilets and backpacker sites of Little Yosemite Valley in just over half a mile. This is the first legal place to set up camp after leaving the valley floor. It's hardly an isolated spot, so be prepared for crowds.

According to park rangers, more than 20 percent of all backcountry campers in Yosemite pass through Little Yosemite Valley. Where there are backpacks laden with delicious snacks, bears soon follow. This area is notorious for bears bold enough to swipe your food off of a stump while you're pitching your tent.

To help manage the impact of so many visitors, rangers have constructed designated fire rings, bear boxes, and composting toilets. Please use these to lessen the effect of high traffic in the backcountry. During the summer months, a ranger lives just east of the campground on the other side of Sunshine Creek; a spur trail to the station departs the JMT shortly after leaving the campground.

After leaving Little Yosemite Valley (6,140 feet), climb moderately for about one hour along the 2.2 miles leading up to the juncture with the Half Dome trail (7,020 feet). If you want to make the

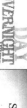

SECTION HIKES

YOSEMITE NATIONAL PARK AND ANSEL ADAMS WILDERNESS

optional 4-mile, 2,000-foot-elevation-gain, round-trip climb (see page 32), leave your pack here. Be sure to stow any food in bear-proof cans and stash your pack out of sight. The likelihood of anyone taking your things is slim, but there's no reason to tempt fate.

From the juncture with the Half Dome trail, continue climbing and within a half mile, pass the trail leading up to Cloud's Rest (7,210 feet). After this point, the scenery opens to sweeping views of the Cascade Cliffs and Bunnell Point, and the trail traffic diminishes. In the mile following the juncture, enter a forested area dotted with red firs and dogwoods along Sunrise Creek. There are a few camp spots here for anyone who wants to avoid the crowds at Little Yosemite Valley. The views here are stupendous as well.

After fording Sunrise Creek, pass through a relatively level wash area often layered with a carpet of wildflowers in the spring and early summer. Enter a lush area with ferns, lupines, and beautiful wild-flowers such as baby blue eyes and columbine along the creek. Shortly thereafter, cross the first of two junctions, one for Merced Lake and a second for the Forsyth Trail. Continue to follow signs for the JMT, fording Sunrise Creek a handful of times. Over the next 4.5 miles, the trail ascends gradually at first, but eventually begins two grueling sets of switchbacks to reach a ridge along Sunrise Mountain with northern views to Cathedral Peak.

Descend the eastern side of the mountain into gorgeous and appropriately named Long Meadow. Early in the season, the mosquitoes can be brutal here, so consider striking camp on a high plateau before descending or continuing past the meadow about a mile past the High Sierra Camp en route to Cathedral Pass.

As you approach the meadow, look for Sunrise High Sierra Camp (9,320 feet), one of five High Sierra Camps that Yosemite offers. The camps are generally spaced 6 to 10 miles apart, where a hot meal, a canvas tent cabin with a bed, and a pack lunch await weary hikers. For more information and current rates and reservations, call

(559) 253-5674 or make reservations online at **www.yosemitepark.com**. Just before you reach the tent cabins, there are a number of backpacker sites that share the fabulous views of the snowcapped peaks of the Clark Range and the namesake sunrises that cast their morning light over the meadow. Backpackers have to forgo hot showers, but composting toilets and bear boxes are located here.

From Sunrise High Sierra Camp, walk along the flat meadow until you reach a junction with the Merced Lake Trail. Begin a gradual ascent up the eastern side of Tresidder Peak, climbing for 30 to 45 minutes to your first view of Echo and Matthes peaks. Another 15 minutes brings you to a stop-worthy panoramic viewing point (9,940 feet) with sun-soaked granite slabs that beckon for a sit and snack. Soak in the splendid grandeur of the Clark Range and the peaks of Tresidder, Cathedral, and Echo.

Drop down to Cathedral Pass (9,700 feet) after rounding the base of Columbia Finger, and then continue your descent through a series of meadows and lakes. In spring, the wildflower display is unbelievable. Upper Cathedral Lake (9,585 feet) is the first in a series of lakes lying in the shadow of their grand namesake. There are some campsites here, but the area is an extremely popular weekend backpacker destination from Tuolumne and can be quite crowded.

Leave the lake and keep descending for 0.75 miles until you pass a sign for Cathedral Lake (Lower Cathedral Lake; 9,288 feet). For a short side trip, follow this spur trail for half a mile through pine woods and along the river to another lovely water jewel in the meadows, perfect for swimming on a blistering day. There are plenty of little bathing nooks along the river as you approach. No camping is allowed at this lower lake.

From the juncture (9,430 feet) with Lower Cathedral Lake, continue downhill on the sandy path to Tuolumne's visitor center (8,630 feet). While it's easy to feel like a horse returning to the barn at this point (or to a cold drink or hot shower), try to savor the granite views and gentle meadows of your descent into Tuolumne. It's a stunning plunge with a few rollers through meadows colored with iris, mountain hemlock, and lodgepole pine woodland. Expect crowded trails, though, packed with day hikers making their way to the lakes.

Arrive at a confusing junction near CA 120. To reach the visitor center, the backpacker's camp, or the continuation of the JMT, turn right and follow signs to the Tuolumne Meadows High Sierra Camp and Glen Aulin. Cross Budd Creek on a footbridge, and at the next juncture either head northward (left) to approach the visitor center or southward (right) to follow signs to the campground.

PERMIT INFORMATION: *To reserve an overnight permit originating in Yosemite, call the Yosemite Wilderness Center at (209) 372-0740 (8:30 a.m. to 4:30 p.m., Monday through Friday), or reserve online at* **www.yosemite.org/visitor/wild.html.** *You can also mail an application to Wilderness Reservations, Yosemite Association, P.O. Box 545, Yosemite, CA 95389. For any of these methods, you will need to provide the following information: your name; address; daytime phone number; number of people in the party; method of travel (foot); number of stock (if applicable); start and end dates; entry and exit trailheads (Happy Isles entry, Tuolumne Meadows exit); principal destination; credit-card number and expiration date, money order, or check for a nonrefundable $5-per-person processing fee.*

If you haven't reserved a permit in advance, you could also try for a walk-in permit at the Yosemite Valley Wilderness Center, located in Yosemite Village next to the post office (open seasonally 9 a.m. to 5 p.m.). About 40 percent of all permits are set aside for walk-ins, but these go quickly during the summer months.

DIRECTIONS: Yosemite can be entered via four main gateways. The BIG OAK FLAT ROAD ENTRANCE is on CA 120 West (Big Oak Flat Road) and is the closest western access to Tuolumne Meadows; the ARCH ROCK ENTRANCE on CA 140 (El Portal Road) is east of Merced and the safest bet in inclement weather, as it receives the least amount of snowfall; the SOUTH ENTRANCE is on CA 41 (Wawona Road), north of Fresno; and the weather-dependent TIOGA PASS ENTRANCE is on CA 120 East (Tioga Road) and is the closest eastern access to Tuolumne Meadows. Tioga Road is closed during the winter months due to snow, and sometimes doesn't open until June or July. While the first three entrances are generally open year-round, all roads are subject to closure; check with the park service by phone at (209) 372-0200 or visit www.nps.gov/yose/planyourvisit/conditions .htm to determine current conditions.

The Happy Isles trailhead is in the southeastern part of Yosemite Valley, 1 mile past Curry Village. Backpackers may leave their cars in the parking lot south of Curry Village near Upper Pines Campground and take the free shuttle bus to Shuttle Stop #16. There is a parking lot at Happy Isles, but it is often full in the summer months.

If you leave a car in Yosemite Valley and need public transit to return to it, YARTS bus service offers a shuttle from Tuolumne Meadows Visitor Center back to the Yosemite Village Visitor Center at 9:10 a.m. during the summer months. Rates are $15 one-way; allow two hours for the journey. Call (888) 89-YARTS or visit www.yarts.com for current rates and schedules.

To drive to Tuolumne Meadows from Happy Isles, head northwest on Big Oak Flat Road for about 30 minutes, then turn right to take Tioga Road (CA 120) about 1 hour through the park to Tuolumne Meadows. This road is closed during snowy conditions. The visitor center parking lot is just off Tioga Road. The park runs a free shuttle-bus service from 7 a.m. to 6:30 p.m. along Tioga Road from Tuolumne Lodge to Olmsted Point from July 4 through Labor Day; the visitor center can be found at Shuttle Stop #6. Tuolumne Meadow can also be accessed via the park's east entrance at Tioga Pass from CA 120, as noted above.

GPS coordinates	*Starting trailhead*	Happy Isles
UTM zone (WGS84)	11S	
Easting	0274558	
Northing	4179230	
Latitude	N 37°43'57.31"	
Longtitude:	W 119°33'31.47"	

GPS coordinates	*Ending trailhead*	Tuolumne
	Meadows Visitor Center	
UTM zone (WGS84)	11S	
Easting	0291463	
Northing	4194284	
Latitude	N 37°52'18.65"	
Longitude	W 119°22'15.81"	

2 Tuolumne Meadows to Red's Meadow

SCENERY: ☆ ☆ ☆ ☆	DISTANCE: *37 miles*
TRAIL CONDITION: ☆ ☆ ☆ ☆	HIKING TIME: *3–5 days*
CHILDREN: ☆ ☆ ☆	OUTSTANDING FEATURES: *Lyell Canyon,*
DIFFICULTY: ☆ ☆ ☆ ☆	*Donahue Pass, Island Pass, Thousand Island Lake,*
SOLITUDE: ☆	*Shadow Lake, Red's Meadow Resort and Campground*

Many thru-hikers begin the John Muir Trail in Tuolumne Meadows, since it's easier to get permits here than from the Happy Isles trailhead. Others start here to avoid the big climb out of Yosemite Valley and enjoy a more manageable trip start. Indeed, this section begins with the flattest expanse of the John Muir Trail: nearly 8 miles of gentle walking along the Lyell Fork of the Tuolumne River through wooded thickets and picture-perfect meadows. Eventually you will tackle Donahue Pass (11,056 feet), home to many enchanting tarns, and Island Pass (10,205 feet), with its unique islets floating at high elevation. The next few days of hiking bring you past lovely alpine lakes with ample camping. Finally, reach the unique geologic formation of Devils Postpile and the relative creature comforts of Red's Meadow, with free hot-spring showers, home-cooked meals, and a general store.

🥾 From the Tuolumne Meadows Visitor Center (8,630 feet), meander east on a level, dusty trail, passing signs for the backpacker's campground and a trailhead for Elizabeth Lake. After 0.5 miles of walking, cross a bridge over the Dana Fork of the Tuolumne River. Shortly thereafter a second bridge takes you over the Lyell Fork. After about 2.5 easy miles, traverse rushing Rafferty Creek on a handsome footbridge (8,720 feet) and begin a beautiful stroll in and out of forest thickets and along the grassy expanse of Lyell Canyon as the trail parallels the Lyell Fork of the Tuolumne River. The area is named for Charles Lyell, a 19th-century lawyer turned geologist and good friend of Charles Darwin.

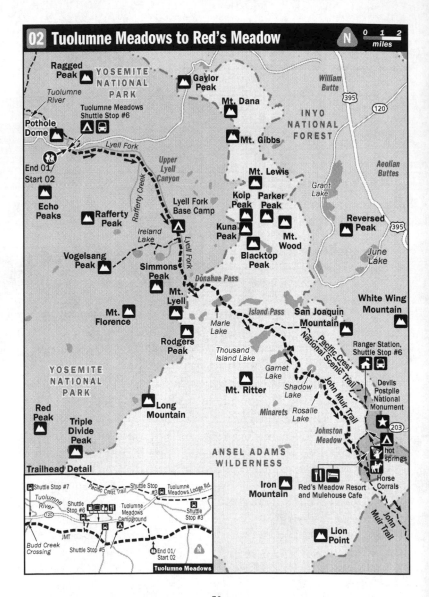

Ragged Peak

YOSEMITE NATIONAL PARK

Gaylor Peak

William Butte

Tuolumne River

Tuolumne Meadows Shuttle Stop #6

Mt. Dana

395

120

Pothole Dome

Lyell Fork

INYO NATIONAL FOREST

Mt. Gibbs

End 01/ Start 02

Upper Lyell Canyon

Rafferty Creek

Mt. Lewis

Aeolian Buttes

Echo Peaks

Rafferty Peak

Koip Peak

Parker Peak

Grant Lake

Ireland Lake

Lyell Fork Base Camp

Kuna Peak

Reversed Peak

395

Vogelsang Peak

Lyell Fork

Mt. Wood

June Lake

Simmons Peak

Donahue Pass

Blacktop Peak

Mt. Lyell

Island Pass

San Joaquin Mountain

White Wing Mountain

Mt. Florence

Marie Lake

Pacific Crest National Scenic Trail

Ranger Station, Shuttle Stop #6

Rodgers Peak

Thousand Island Lake

Garnet Lake

John Muir Trail

Devils Postpile National Monument

YOSEMITE NATIONAL PARK

Mt. Ritter

Shadow Lake

203

Red Peak

Long Mountain

Minarets

Rosalie Lake

Johnston Meadow

hot springs

Triple Divide Peak

Horse Corrals

ANSEL ADAMS WILDERNESS

Iron Mountain

Red's Meadow Resort and Mulehouse Cafe

John Muir Trail

Trailhead Detail

Shuttle Stop #7

Pacific Crest Trail

Shuttle Stop #3

Tuolumne Meadows Lodge Rd.

Tuolumne River

Shuttle Stop #6

120

Tuolumne Meadows Campground

Shuttle Stop #3

JMT

Budd Creek Crossing

Shuttle Stop #5

End 01/ Start 02

N

Lion Point

Tuolumne Meadows

Up until the mid-1800s and the explosion of silver prospectors and explorers, only Native Americans enjoyed the beauty of this region. Miwok and Mono Indians stopped in the area to trade during the summer en route east. These days, though, visitors from around the world come to marvel at the landscape. Rainbow trout lure anglers to this stretch of Yosemite from late April through mid-November.

The trail's proximity to busy Tuolumne Meadows, as well as its level grade, nearly guarantees that you will have company in this part of the wilderness. The presence of hikers careless with their food, combined with shallow waters teeming with fish, also means that this is popular bear and deer country. Be sure to keep your snacks and food secure at all times. Camping is prohibited within the first 4 miles from Tuolumne Meadows. Bear canisters are essential here, and there is no question that you will lose your food if you don't have one.

After crossing Rafferty Creek, reach the next trail junction in a little more than 4 miles at the turnoff (8,900 feet) for Ireland Lake, savoring views of the Unicorn and Mammoth peaks along the way. Shortly after passing this trail juncture, encounter Potter Point and numerous campsites. Ahead, glimpse Mount Lyell, the park's highest peak at 13,114 feet, and Donahue Pass beckoning in the distance.

ELEVATION PROFILE

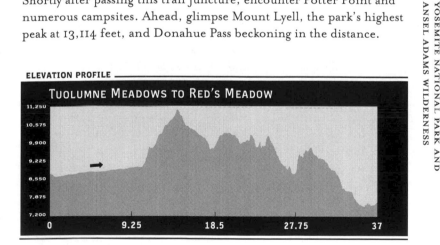

TUOLUMNE MEADOWS TO RED'S MEADOW

About 8 miles from the visitor center, the trail turns away from the river and begins the initial climb toward Donahue Pass, passing a well-used camping area. Dubbed Lyell Fork Base Camp (9,040 feet), this area is popular with local backpackers and sees quite a bit of use in the summer months. Initially the climb is in a shaded pine bench, and then it evolves into steeper exposed switchbacks with fantastic views back toward the valley. After 1.5 miles, the trail flattens for a bit and reaches a bridge over the Lyell Fork (9,650 feet). There are camping sites on either side of this sturdy footbridge. After crossing the river, begin climbing again, sometimes quite steeply, up a rocky set of switchbacks. Your prize is a stunning mountain tarn (10,200 feet) surrounded by meadows and nestled in a cirque at the base of Donahue Pass. There are a few camping spots here scattered amid the whitebark pines should you arrive in the late afternoon and wish to conquer Donahue Pass (11,056 feet) in the morning.

From the lakelet, cross the southern stream outlet to resume climbing. Often this crossing requires knee-deep wading in the early months of the hiking season (June and July, particularly). Continue up a series of granite switchbacks until reaching a second tarn. This is desolate country, beautiful in its barren shale and scrub. Traverse this plateau and cross the next small lake's outlet. In early spring, it's likely you will encounter a snowfield crossing before beginning the final shale and rock ascent toward the pass. Remember to keep looking back for epic views of Yosemite Valley.

The pass itself is a little undefined, and often the sign marking it has been trampled by the winter's snow. Arrival is assured, however, by the stunning view of the alpine wilderness, including the Mount Ritter range, which stretches out ahead. This is where you must say good-bye to Yosemite, as you amble into the Inyo National Forest and Ansel Adams Wilderness. Formerly called the Minarets Wilderness, the area was renamed in 1984 to honor the famous photographer and environmentalist.

Descend 3.5 miles eastward through a barren landscape of granite rocks and stark tarns with stately Banner Peak luring you closer. Descending to 9,600 feet, the granite slabs give way to an idyllic landscape of forests, alpine lakes, and rampant wildflowers. Many times you'll ford Rush Creek, which, depending on the season, can be a shoes-off affair. The most difficult crossing comes just before the junction (10,030 feet) with the Marie Lakes Trail, 3 miles from the crest of Donahue Pass. En route, enjoy wonderful views of the Ritter range and the jagged spires of the Minarets. Legend has it that the spires served as the backdrop for the Wicked Witch of the West's home in the original film version of *The Wizard of Oz*.

Continuing down, enter the Rush Creek Forks area, and the junction for the Rush Creek Trail. Follow and ford the creek before beginning a gradual 1.5-mile ascent toward Island Pass (10,205 feet), with its incredibly picturesque high alpine lakes and meadows. It's a bit difficult to determine exactly where the pass's highest point is, as the climb plateaus out among many gorgeous lakelets.

Tear yourself away from the splendid pass and descend toward Thousand Island Lake (9,833 feet), named for the myriad islets floating within its boundaries. If the stunning view of Banner Peak reflected in the water feels familiar, that's because it has graced many of Ansel Adams's visually arresting black-and-white photos. A San Francisco native and renowned photographer and environmentalist, Adams joined the Sierra Club at the age of 17 and began climbing these same mountains shortly thereafter. Within this section of the wilderness named for him, it's nearly impossible to take a bad picture. Camping is not permitted within a quarter mile of the lake's outlets, but there are a few well-positioned sites on the lake's northwest flank.

As you round the lake, the John Muir Trail (JMT) and Pacific Crest Trail (PCT) part ways, not reuniting again until Devils Postpile National Monument. The JMT continues across a log bridge over the lake's outlet, while the PCT turns to travel the High Trail over the San Joaquin Mountains. Our route follows the JMT.

After a mild descent, the trail rolls upward toward gorgeous Emerald Lake, your first in a series of gem-named lakes. Just past Emerald is Ruby Lake, with good camping on its northern shore. Ascend to Ruby Ridge and drop down a series of switchbacks to Garnet Lake (9,678 feet), a miniature version of Thousand Island Lake with its many islets and picture-perfect backdrop of Mount Ritter and Banner Peak. As with all the lakes, you can't camp within a quarter mile of their outlets, but there are a few campsites flanking the northwest shores. On a mosquito-laden day, Garnet's constant wind provides welcome relief from the bloodsucking beasts; the wind, though, can be a bit chilly in colder seasons. This is a favored spot for backcountry anglers and Boy Scouts, so solitude is not likely.

Cross a picturesque footbridge, ignoring the unmarked trail that joins from the left, begin climbing, skirt the lake's southeastern shore, then ascend steeply. Just before reaching the top of the saddle, look for a small pool for cooling off with a quick dip—highly recommended. Next, enjoy a long rocky descent, often with little water available in the mid to late season. It's a bit of a knee buster as you approach the creek. Cross the Shadow Creek footbridge and approach Shadow Lake (8,737 feet). The JMT skirts the lake on the south side, while the trail leading out to Agnew Meadow trailhead (4 miles from this juncture) skirts around its northern side.

Follow the southern shore of luscious Shadow Lake. To cool down, a quick swim is encouraged before the climb resumes. The perfectly graded switchbacks that lead up from Shadow Lake make the almost 700-foot climb much easier than most; your knees will appreciate the dirt trail, as opposed to granite boulders, and the shade of fragrant pine trees is helpful. It's a nice steady walk up to Rosalie Lake (9,350 feet), where the trail levels briefly, allowing hikers a respite from climbing. This is a popular weekend destination from Red's

Meadow, and there are many campgrounds (and campers!) here. The climbing isn't quite over yet, with one last hump up to shallow Gladys Lake (9,580 feet). While not that much of a climb, it can feel like it after a long day. There is camping here as well.

To continue, begin a seemingly endless downhill of more than 2,000 feet to Red's Meadow. The dusty trail passes through pine trees, with only the occasional mountain tarns of Trinity Lakes (9,180 feet) breaking up the descent. At long last, reach the welcome junction of Johnston Meadows and Lake (8,120 feet) and enter Devils Postpile National Monument. This national monument is named for its unique and rare set of basalt columns, which rise 60 feet into the air with eerie geometric consistency. The columns resulted from the cooling and shrinking of lava flows and are thought to be less than 100,000 years old—relatively new by geological standards. For more information on the formations and day hikes in the area, see page 48.

Signposts along the following segment can be confusing. Follow signs to Devils Postpile and walk through this area (with a final climb!) until reaching the junction with Red's Meadow, where the PCT rejoins the trail. From here, there are a number of options: The first way to reach civilization is to continue straight toward Devils Postpile, veer left at the next junction, cross the bridge, and veer left again to hike out to the ranger station at Devils Postpile Campground. This is Shuttle Stop #6. A free bus runs here seasonally from 7:30 a.m. to 6:20 p.m., and it can take you to Red's Meadow Resort (Shuttle Stop #10), a short distance from the Red's Meadow Campground. You can also shuttle from here all the way to Mammoth Mountain Inn. See the Directions for more transit information.

Otherwise, to continue walking to Red's Meadow, instead of veering left at the second intersection toward the ranger station, follow signs to Devils Postpile, John Muir Trail South, and Red's Meadow, passing in front of the basalt columns to the next junction. To bypass the campground and head directly to Red's Meadow Resort from here, turn right to follow the trail to the amenities at Red's. For the campground, walk straight toward the road, turn left, then cross the street to follow a path into the camp. At the campground, there is a free walk-in site for backpackers on your left. It can get crowded (and even full!), but it's usually a friendly and accommodating crowd. The highlight for most at Red's Meadow Campground is the free hot-spring-fed showers (bathhouse). You'll find the naturally heated showers at the top of the campground, near the restrooms. You can also just follow the slight smell of sulfur and the long line of hikers waiting with towels.

The trail to Red's Meadow Resort and the return to the JMT is directly across from the restrooms near the showers and bathhouse. This short path to the resort is surprisingly lovely considering its proximity to the road. Look for aspens, horsetail ferns, and vibrant wildflowers scattered about the hillside rising toward the resort.

Those looking for food caches can collect them at the Red's Meadow Resort's general store (mid-June through mid-September; 7 a.m. to 7 p.m.), while those looking for a hot meal can step into the Mulehouse Café (mid-June through mid-September; 7 a.m. to 7 p.m.). There is also a hiker's barrel at the back of the general store, where hikers can leave food they don't want and scavenge for a little upgrade to their culinary assortment. It sometimes includes clothing and gear.

If you're planning a layover day at Red's Meadow, consider doing a day hike to Rainbow Falls and further exploring Devils Postpile National Monument. For more information, see page 48.

PERMIT INFORMATION: *To reserve an overnight permit originating in Yosemite, call the Yosemite Wilderness Center at (209) 372-0740 (8:30 a.m. to 4:30 p.m., Monday through Friday), or reserve online at* **www.yosemite.org/visitor/wild.html.** *You can also mail an application to Wilderness Reservations, Yosemite Association, P.O. Box 545, Yosemite, CA 95389. For any of these methods, you will need to provide the following information: your name; address; daytime phone number;*

number of people in the party; method of travel (foot); number of stock (if applicable); start and end dates; entry and exit trailheads (Tuolumne Meadows entry, Red's Meadow exit); principal destination; credit-card number and expiration date, money order, or check for a nonrefundable $5-per-person processing fee.

If you haven't reserved a permit in advance, you could also try for a walk-in permit at the Tuolumne Meadows Wilderness Center, located off Tioga Road in the parking lot before the Tuolumne Lodge (open seasonally 9 a.m. to 5 p.m.). About 40 percent of all permits are set aside for walk-ins, but these go quickly during the summer months.

DIRECTIONS: TUOLUMNE MEADOWS CAMPGROUND—Yosemite can be entered via four main gateways: The BIG OAK FLAT ROAD ENTRANCE is on CA 120 West (Big Oak Flat Road) and is the closest western access to Tuolumne Meadows; the ARCH ROCK ENTRANCE on CA 140 (El Portal Road) is east of Merced and the safest bet in inclement weather, as it receives the least amount of snowfall; the SOUTH ENTRANCE is on CA 41 (Wawona Road), north of Fresno; and the weather-dependent TIOGA PASS ENTRANCE is on CA 120 East (Tioga Road); it is the closest eastern access point to Tuolumne Meadows. Tioga Road is closed during the winter months due to snow, and sometimes doesn't open until June or July. While the first three entrances are generally open year-round, all roads are subject to closure; check with the park service by phone at (209) 372-0200 or visit www.nps.gov/yose/plan yourvisit/conditions.htm to determine current conditions. Tuolumne Meadows is in the eastern area of Yosemite National Park off Tioga Road (CA 120 East). For parking, follow signs to the Tuolumne Lodge and Wilderness Permit office. There is a parking lot on the left sign-posted for Dog Lake and the John Muir Trail, or you may find additional parking in the Wilderness Permit lot and then follow the signs to the John Muir Trail. The park runs a free shuttle-bus service from 7 a.m. to 6:30 p.m. along Tioga Road from Tuolumne Lodge to Olmsted Point from July 4 through Labor Day; the trailhead can be found at Shuttle Stop #2.

RED'S MEADOW CAMPGROUND—Red's Meadow can be reached from Mammoth Lakes. From the Mammoth Ranger Station and Visitor Center (on CA 203, 3 miles west of US 395), head west on Main Street for 1.5 miles and turn right to continue on CA 203 (Minaret Road), climbing nearly 5 miles to Mammoth Mountain Inn.

During the summer months, you cannot access Red's Meadow or the Devils Postpile National Monument via car from 7 a.m. to 7:30 p.m. unless you have campground or resort reservations, a handicap placard, or a special permit. Wilderness Permits do not allow you vehicular access. Mandatory shuttles operate from the parking area in front of Mammoth Mountain Inn beginning at 7:15 a.m. Tickets can be purchased at the Gondola Building in the Main Lodge; the 45-minute shuttle to the Devils Postpile area is free for kids under 3, $4 for children ages 3 to 15, and $7 for all other adults. Shuttle service within the national-monument area between campgrounds and trailheads is free; Red's Meadow Resort and Campground is Shuttle Stop #10. For more information, contact the Mammoth Ranger Station and Visitor Center at (760) 924-5500 or visit the city's regional-transit site at www.ci.mammothlakes.ca.us/transit/regional_transit.htm.

If you have reservations or are traveling in the off-season (October through early June), continue driving up the hill to the Minaret Summit Entrance Station (9,175 feet) and follow the steep narrow road the remaining 7 miles to the Devils Postpile Monument Area, Red's Meadow, trailheads, and campgrounds.

For hikers not being picked up at Red's Meadow, you may also return to Yosemite from Mammoth via public transit on the YARTS bus. Buses leave from various points in Mammoth to Tuolumne once daily between 7 a.m. to 7:30 a.m. ($20; about two hours each way). Call (888) 89-YARTS or visit www.yarts.com for current rates and schedules. Unfortunately, because the shuttle bus that leaves Red's Meadow for Mammoth does not arrive early enough for visitors to catch the bus back to Yosemite, you'll have to overnight in Mammoth in a hotel or RV campground.

Public transit is also available to Mammoth Lakes along US 395 between Reno and Ridgecrest via Inyo Mono Transit's CREST bus. The bus travels north between Bishop and Reno via Mammoth Lakes on Tuesday, Thursday, and Friday, and south between Mammoth Lakes and Ridgecrest on Monday, Wednesday, and Friday. There is also limited Saturday service between Bishop and Mammoth lakes only. Rates and routes are subject to frequent change; call ahead for information and reservations at (760) 872-1901 or (800) 922-1930. More information can be found on the Web at www.countyofinyo.org/transit/CRESTpage.htm.

To take advantage of these public-transit options, you must travel between Mammoth Mountain Inn, where the Red's Meadow Shuttle drops you, and the city of Mammoth Lakes, from which the CREST and YARTS buses depart. This can be done via the Bike Park Shuttle that operates from 9 a.m. to 5:30 p.m. daily, late June through September. The bike shuttle runs from the Mammoth Lakes Village transportation hub (Minaret Road at Canyon Boulevard) to the Adventure Center located across the street from Mammoth Mountain Inn. This service is free for hikers. It's important to note, however, that if you catch the last bus (7:45 p.m.) out of Red's Meadow toward Mammoth Mountain Inn, you will need to hitchhike the final 4 miles to Mammoth Lakes.

Lastly, you could contact Mammoth Shuttle by phone at (760) 934-6588 to arrange for private transit on demand. This is a pricey option but may be worth it for larger groups. Prices range considerably from $100 (from one eastern-Sierra trailhead to another) to $600 (from Mammoth to Kings Canyon). The price to go from Mammoth to Yosemite averages $200 (per eight-passenger shuttle, not per person).

GPS coordinates	*Starting trailhead* Tuolumne Meadows Wilderness Permit Center
UTM zone (WGS84)	11S
Easting	0293669
Northing	4194684
Latitude	N 37°52'33.15"
Longitude	W 119°20'59.53"

GPS coordinates	*Ending trailhead* Red's Meadow Campground
UTM zone (WGS84)	11S
Easting	0316834
Northing	4165592
Latitude	N 37°37'9.14"
Longitude	W 119°04'21.91"

Ansel Adams Wilderness and John Muir Wilderness

RED'S MEADOW, VERMILION RESORT, FLORENCE LAKE

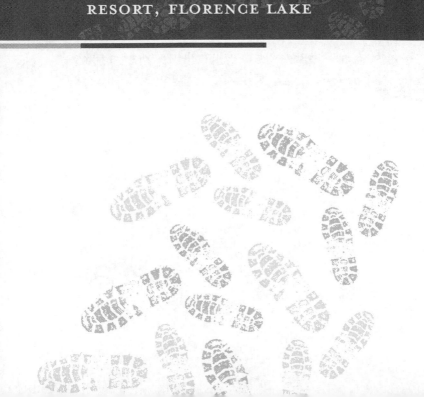

In the high altitude, you soar above the treeline with wide granite expanses and endless views. In lower elevations, relish the rich diversity of flora in sunny meadows and shady forest thickets. Throughout, find a range of lakes, streams, rivers, and distinct ecosystems

3 Red's Meadow to Vermilion Valley Resort

SCENERY: ✿ ✿ ✿ ✿	DISTANCE: *31 miles*
TRAIL CONDITION: ✿ ✿ ✿ ✿	HIKING TIME: *3–5 days*
CHILDREN: ✿ ✿	OUTSTANDING FEATURES: *Red Cones,*
DIFFICULTY: ✿ ✿ ✿	*Purple Lake, Lake Virginia, Squaw Lake, Silver Pass,*
SOLITUDE: ✿ ✿	*Pocket Meadow, Edison Lake Ferry*

This section travels from the relative creature comforts of one backcountry refuge to another. You'd be wise to enjoy this pampering as the trail becomes increasingly more remote as it meanders south. From Red's Meadow, it's a long, hot, and sometimes exposed climb through an area ravaged by 1992's Rainbow Fire. However Purple and Virginia lakes provide the perfect setting for a high-altitude swim to wash off any trail dust. Enjoy a tremendous descent into Tully Hole and walk along the banks of Fish Creek, rolling up toward Squaw Lake. Silver Pass (10,895 feet) is the most significant climb of this stretch, affording epic views of Cascade Valley. From here, it's virtually all downhill as the trail wanders through Pocket Meadow before descending to Lake Edison. Hop on a ferry that whisks you away to cold beer and hot food at the Vermilion Valley Resort. The "resort" part is a bit of a stretch—it's no Four Seasons— but they've got tent cabins, showers, and great eats.

🚶🚶 From Red's Meadow Resort (7,600 feet), the John Muir Trail (JMT) isn't initially clear: To access the route, walk through the horse corrals and continue southeast on the unmarked trail. Within a quarter mile reach a sign for the Pacific Crest Trail (PCT) and shortly thereafter follow the route marked to Red Cones.

Traverse the wide, dusty basin through manzanita, aspen trees, and waist-high ferns, noting the havoc wreaked by the Rainbow Fire. Named for nearby waterfalls, the blaze swept through the region in 1992, scarring close to 8,000 acres in its lightning-induced wake. Now the remaining tree snags provide excellent roosts for an abundance of birds, including the brightly coated Western Tanager. The opened

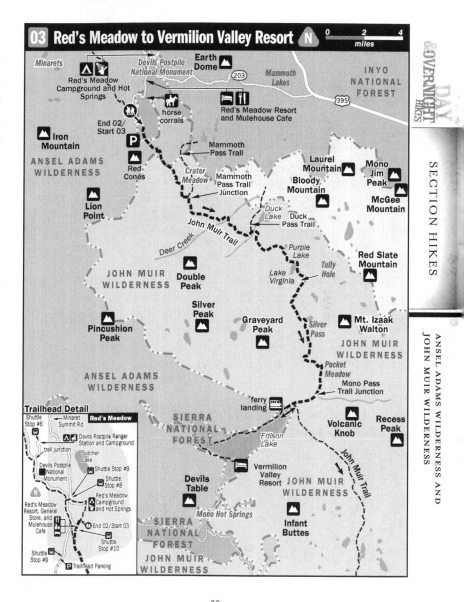

03 Red's Meadow to Vermilion Valley Resort

N

0   2   4
miles

Minarets

Red's Meadow Campground and Hot Springs

Earth Dome

Devils Postpile National Monument

(203)

Mammoth Lakes

INYO NATIONAL FOREST

395

Red's Meadow Resort and Mulehouse Cafe

horse corrals

End 02/ Start 03

P

Iron Mountain

ANSEL ADAMS WILDERNESS

Red Cones

Mammoth Pass Trail

Crater Meadow

Mammoth Pass Trail Junction

Laurel Mountain

Bloody Mountain

Mono Jim Peak

McGee Mountain

Lion Point

John Muir Trail

Deer Creek

Duck Lake

Duck Pass Trail

JOHN MUIR WILDERNESS

Double Peak

Purple Lake

Lake Virginia

Tully Hole

Red Slate Mountain

Silver Peak

Graveyard Peak

Silver Pass

Mt. Izaak Walton

Pincushion Peak

ANSEL ADAMS WILDERNESS

JOHN MUIR WILDERNESS

Pocket Meadow

Mono Pass Trail Junction

ferry landing

Volcanic Knob

Recess Peak

Trailhead Detail

Shuttle Stop #6

Minaret Summit Rd.

Red's Meadow

Devils Postpile Ranger Station and Campground

trail junction

Sotcher Lake

Shuttle Stop #9

Devils Postpile National Monument

Shuttle Stop #8

Red's Meadow Campground and Hot Springs

Red's Meadow Resort, General Store, and Mulehouse Cafe

End 02/Start 03

Shuttle Stop #10

Shuttle Stop #9

Trailhead Parking

SIERRA NATIONAL FOREST

Edison Lake

Devils Table

Mono Hot Springs

Vermilion Valley Resort

JOHN MUIR WILDERNESS

SIERRA NATIONAL FOREST

JOHN MUIR WILDERNESS

John Muir Trail

Infant Buttes

canopy, dotted with lodgepole pines, allows for a greater diversity of ground cover and a fiery display of wildflowers. Consider wearing pants on the first stretch of this trail, as the low foliage is narrow, dense, and somewhat scratchy.

Begin climbing a series of switchbacks under the welcome shade of more mature trees ascending above the fire zone. Cross several small branches of Boundary Creek before rising to the lovely plateau below Crater Meadow, where Indian paintbrush, asters, and monkey flower abound. Continue rising along the sandy, pumice-laden trail and enjoy views of the backside of Mammoth Mountain.

A dormant volcano, Mammoth lies on the rim of Long Valley Caldera, a region that is known as one of the Sierra's "hot spots" due to ever-present geothermal activity. Ironic, considering that Mammoth is a mecca for snow sports in the winter. Considered young, as it was formed by numerous eruptions between 220,000 and 50,000 years ago, Mammoth is part of the same magmatic chain as the Red Cones, volcanic cinder cones named for their rich red color. The reddish hue is a result of scoria deposits on their mantle, and carbon dating places the unglaciated cones at just under 9,000 years old.

A side trail to Mammoth Pass veers off to your left (northeast) shortly before you cross Crater Creek (8,920 feet) and leave Ansel

ELEVATION PROFILE

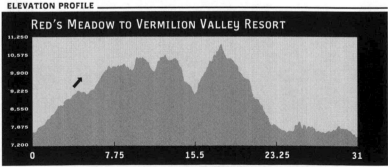

Adams Wilderness to enter John Muir Wilderness. Walk a short spell along an idyllic creek lined by fir trees and lupine, and come through a shady plateau into gorgeous Upper Crater Meadow. Red's Meadow now lies 4 miles away. Traverse a few streams on raised earthen bridges before entering the woods and resuming a moderate climb. Reach popular campsites at the crossing of Deer Creek (9,150 feet). Be sure to load up on water here, as the next water source lies nearly 6 miles away at Duck Creek.

Resume ascending gently in the shade of trees. Rising closer to 10,000 feet, stunning views of the Silver Divide mountains reveal themselves through the conifers to your right. Rounding the ridge above Cascade Valley, drop down toward Duck Creek, noticing a number of popular campsites as you approach the ford of Duck Lake's outlet. Flat tent sites can be found on either side of the creek.

After the Duck Lake outlet crossing, begin mounting a series of rocky exposed switchbacks. Mule trains are not uncommon here as they travel to the pack station at Red's Meadow. Ignore a side trail to Duck Pass veering off to the left before reaching the top of the saddle (10,460 feet), and follow signs to Purple Lake. Walk along a sandy ridge, moderately shaded with pine trees, and enjoy sweeping views over Cascade Valley to the snow-capped mountains beyond. Begin dropping toward Purple Lake with manzanita lining the rocky path.

Purple Lake (9,928 feet) sits in an exquisite tree-lined cirque. There is great camping here, although it's popular with stock horses and mule trains, so less private than other areas. After skirting the lake on the southern shore, ignore a sign to Marsh Lake and follow a subsequent JMT sign, crossing a wooden bridge over the lake's outlet and begin climbing again. The switchbacks from Purple Lake are superbly well engineered, albeit not effortless. The first bit is intermittently shaded, but then there's a long exposed section that can be brutal in the hot sun. Reach a high point at 10,500 feet, for fabulous vistas and the whirring sound of dragonflies, before dropping down moderately toward Lake Virginia (10,338 feet). The lake is dazzling, but also very exposed and frequently quite windy; making it great for keeping the mosquitoes at bay but a bit chilly for swimming. There are some exposed campsites here. Continuing on, the outlet can be difficult to cross, but well-placed rocks should guide the way amid a field of vibrant Indian paintbrush.

Switchback up, skirting the lake's northeast shore, and continue past reddish granite rocks tumbling toward the shore. Traverse a rather flat, sandy wash section before beginning a dizzying descent toward Tully Hole (9,520 feet). Long, exposed, vertigo-inducing zigzags lead to the meadow below with expansive views ever present. At the bottom, follow rushing Fish Creek as it tumbles over rocks. There are plenty of places to camp along here.

Ignore McGee Pass junction and continue following signs to Silver Pass. Cross a steel footbridge to find more camping sites and the junction with the Cascade Valley Trail. Continue straight and begin ascending up the shady path toward Silver Pass. It's a long climb, continually along the creek, with lush wooded sections and several creek fords. Water is plentiful, and the canyon is dark and moist with intermittent campsites. The path steepens just below the upper rocky basin that cradles Squaw Lake. Climb nicely cut granite stairs and enjoy marvelous backward views. Squaw Lake (10,300 feet) sits nestled in a dramatic granite amphitheater. There are a few scrubby pines amid the grass and a handful of exposed campsites with stellar sunset views. Cross the lake's northwestern outlet to continue climbing. It's 1.5 miles and 600 feet of ascension from here to the top of Silver Pass.

Climb 300 feet to junction with Goodale Pass Trail and the Lake of the Lone Indian. The scenery is spartan and expansive, and it's possible to camp here. Keep climbing until the trail plateaus a bit near Chief Lake set among scrubby boulders and tarns and cradled by grand craggy mountains. Catch your breath before the next series of switchbacks and admire the views back toward Papoose Lake.

Approach the pass through an exposed broad cirque. Much of the year the final push to grand Silver Pass (10,900 feet) requires traversing a snowfield.

You may notice that the snow has a pinkish hue. The Sierra Nevada range is well known for its high-altitude "watermelon snow," a phenomenon resulting from an algae bloom that thrives in cold temperatures. The scientific term is *Chlamydomonas nivalis,* and if you compress the snow under your boot or make snowballs, the reddish tint is heightened. Despite the sweetish watermelon scent from which the snow derives its name, it is ill-advised to taste the pink snow, as it's rumored to cause severe gastrointestinal issues. As a general rule, it's best to never eat colored snow—pink, yellow, or otherwise!

To truly appreciate the view from the pass, climb the higher rocks to the western side of the pass and soak in an eyeful of breathtaking snowcapped mountains and lakes. Essentially, it's all downhill from here, more than 3,000 feet, all the way to Edison Ferry, 8.5 miles away. Say good-bye to the Inyo National Forest and descend into Sierra National Forest on the southern side of the pass.

Hike down past the gorgeous turquoise waters of an unnamed mountain tarn, where there is little to no camping, and continue through boulder-strewn grasslands to lovely Silver Pass Lake, to find several fine campsites. This is very exposed country with little shade but tremendous views.

The descent moves from open exposed area to wooded meadow and finally down precipitous switchbacks to the North Fork Mono Creek. Continue down, down, down steep and loose rock. The final descent toward the river can be a bit of a knee buster, with two challenging fords that require caution: one at Silver Pass Creek and the other over the North Fork Mono Creek. After crossing the river this second time, continue descending and ignore the trail to Mott Lake. The JMT skirts briefly away from the water to enter shady Pocket Meadow, where campsites are plentiful.

Enjoy a more moderate descent along the creek, and meander through waist-high monkey flower and grasses dotted with Yosemite asters and black-eyed Susans. Water tumbles over smooth slabs of granite, and sunlit meadows give way intermittently to aspen groves and wooded thickets. As the view opens up, begin switchbacking down again, ignoring the Mono Creek Trail and continuing to follow signs to Selden Pass. After this juncture, the trail becomes nearly flat. Cross the river and walk through shaded stands of cool pine trees with a few gentle rises thrown in to break up the monotony of the descent.

At the juncture in Quail Meadows, a trail to the left heads across a bridge to continue on the JMT toward Selden Pass. Instead, leave the JMT briefly and head straight toward Edison Lake. Relatively flat and shady, the trail uses wooden plankways to protect the more fragile grasslands. Continue 1.4 miles to reach another juncture. The trail straight ahead travels the 4.8 miles to Vermilion Valley Resort, skirting the northwestern shore of Lake Edison. Most hikers, however, choose to turn left and walk another quarter mile to reach the ferry landing (7,720 feet). En route, pass camp spots and lots of good slabs for sunning or lunching, with water cascading over the rocks.

Ferries depart from this landing from June 1 to October 1 (seasonally dependent on snowpack) at 9:45 a.m. and 4:45 p.m. for the 20-minute journey. Regular rates are $10 one-way, $15 round-trip, although private ferry trips can be arranged in advance through Vermilion Valley Resort. There is decent swimming near the northern outlet that feeds into Edison Lake if you have to wait a while. Sometimes this area is choked with fishermen, but it's invariably a friendly crowd, and a great place to wash off the trail dust before reaching the relative oasis of great food, cold beer, hot showers, laundry facilities, and general merriment of Vermilion Valley Resort.

Vermilion Valley Resort (VVR) was established in 1994 by Butch and Peggy Wiggs. It quickly became known as a home away from home for JMT and PCT thru-hikers. While, sadly, Butch passed away in 2001, the resort has retained its open-armed welcome to the weary and dirty that find their way to its rustic charm. Indeed, they still offer a free bed and a beverage to all thru-hikers, along with one of the lowest rates for their food-cache storage and delivery (see page 21 for more information on sending food).

The general method is to start a tab at the front desk of the sundries store. Put all your meals, showers, laundry, phone usage, ferry tickets, and beverages on a tab and then pay with plastic or cash before you leave. Be forewarned, however, that your tab can add up quickly! The general store has a small selection of vital items (food, sunscreen, bug spray, bandages, ponchos, fishing gear, iodine tablets for water purification), but it's no full-blown equipment store. There is a scale outside the store to weigh your pack—and many load theirs up for bragging rights here.

Loud and friendly, VVR is not necessarily a place of restful solitude, but for many it's the perfect antidote to many miles spent hiking the quiet backcountry. Campfires, drunken sing-alongs, and newfound friends are de rigueur. There is also a frequently picked-through hiker's barrel with up-for-grabs food and clothing that other hikers have unloaded or donated. If there are no tent cabins available, simply pitch a tent in what they have dubbed "Sherwood Forest," essentially the patch of dirt and trees in front of the parking area. It may not be the most beautiful spot you've ever camped, but it's within stumbling distance of the flush toilets, showers, and restaurant, and most are happy to call it home.

The most memorable aspect of VVR is hands-down their fantastic food—homemade pie, rib-sticking barbecue, and always a veggie option for any noncarnivores. Befitting with the eclectic character of the place, their chef had a prior life as a tenured philosophy professor at UC Berkeley before switching gears and enrolling in culinary school.

PERMIT INFORMATION: *Permits that originate in the Inyo National Forest can be reserved by contacting the Wilderness Permit Reservation Office (351 Pacu Lane, Suite 200, Bishop, CA 93514), open 8 a.m. to 4:30 p.m. daily from June 1 to October 1 and Monday through Friday during the rest of the year. You can reserve over the phone at (760) 873-2483, by fax at (760) 873-2484, or by mail. You will need to provide the following information: your name; address; daytime phone number; number of people in the party; method of travel (foot); number of stock (if applicable); start and end dates; entry and exit trailheads (Red's Meadow entry, Lake Edison exit); principal destination; credit-card number and expiration date, money order, or check for a nonrefundable $5-per-person processing fee.*

You can then pick up your permit at the Mammoth Lakes Wilderness Permit Office and Visitor Center (2500 Main Street, Mammoth Lakes, CA 93546). Office hours are 8 a.m. to 5 p.m., but if you call ahead they can put your permit in the box outside the office for pickup if you are arriving late.

About 60 percent of permits are reservable; the remainder are set aside for walk-in permits. You can get a walk-in permit at the Mammoth Lakes Wilderness Permit Office and Visitor Center as well as at Devils Postpile Ranger Station, 9 a.m. to 5 p.m.; phone (760) 934-2289.

DIRECTIONS: RED'S MEADOW RESORT—**Red's Meadow can be reached from Mammoth Lakes. From the Mammoth Ranger Station and Visitor Center (on CA 203, 3 miles west of US 395), head west on Main Street for 1.5 miles and turn right to continue on CA 203 (Minaret Road), climbing nearly 5 miles to Mammoth Mountain Inn.**

During the summer months, you cannot access Red's Meadow or the Devils Postpile National Monument via car from 7 a.m. to 7:30 p.m. unless you have campground or resort reservations, a handicap placard, or a special permit. Wilderness Permits do not allow you vehicular access. Mandatory shuttles operate from the parking area in front of Mammoth Mountain Inn beginning at 7:15 a.m. Tickets can be purchased at the Gondola Building in the Main Lodge; the 45-minute shuttle to the Devils Postpile area is free for children

under age 3, $4 for children ages 3 to 15, and $7 for adults. Shuttle service within the national-monument area between campgrounds and trailheads is free; Red's Meadow Resort and Campground is Shuttle Stop #10. For more information, contact the Mammoth Ranger Station and Visitor Center at (760) 924-5500 or visit www.ci.mammoth-lakes.ca.us/transit/regional_transit.htm.

If you have reservations or are traveling in the off-season (October to early June), continue driving up the hill to the Minaret Summit Entrance Station (9,175 feet) and follow the steep, narrow road the remaining 7 miles to the Devils Postpile Monument Area, Red's Meadow, trailheads, and campgrounds.

Public transit is available to Mammoth Lakes along US 395 between Reno and Ridgecrest via Inyo Mono Transit's CREST bus. The bus travels north between Bishop and Reno via Mammoth Lakes on Tuesday, Thursday, and Friday, and south between Mammoth Lakes and Ridgecrest on Monday, Wednesday, and Friday. There is also limited Saturday service between Bishop and Mammoth Lakes only. Rates and routes are subject to frequent change; call ahead for information and reservations at (760) 872-1901 or (800) 922-1930. More information can be found on the Web at www.countyofinyo.org/transit/CRESTpage.htm.

Public transit also services the route between Yosemite and Mammoth Lakes. YARTS buses leave from various points in Yosemite to Mammoth Lakes once daily between 5 p.m. and 6:50 p.m. ($15; approximately two hours each way). Contact YARTS at (888) 89-YARTS or visit www.yarts.com for current rates and schedules. This does, however, force an overnight in Mammoth Lakes.

To take advantage of these public-transit options, you must travel the 4 miles between Mammoth Mountain Inn, where the Red's Meadow Shuttle drops you, and the city of Mammoth Lakes, from which the CREST and YARTS buses depart. This can be done via the Bike Park Shuttle that operates from 9 a.m. to 5:30 p.m. daily, late June through September. The bike shuttle runs from the Mammoth Lakes Village transportation hub (Minaret Road at Canyon Boulevard) to the Adventure Center located across the street from Mammoth Mountain Inn. This service is free for hikers.

Lastly, you could contact Mammoth Shuttle by phone at (760) 934-6588 to arrange for private transit on demand. This is a pricey option but may be worth it for larger groups. Prices range considerably from $100 (from one eastern-Sierra trailhead to another) to $600 (from Mammoth to Kings Canyon). The price to go from Mammoth to Yosemite averages $200 (per eight-passenger shuttle, not per person).

VERMILION VALLEY RESORT—To get to Vermilion Valley Resort (VVR), you will most likely need a friend to pick you up or try your hand at hitchhiking. The closest main highway is CA 168, 30 miles northeast of Fresno, but the final 14 to 20 miles of your journey is a feat to be applauded. VVR even makes a T-shirt that boasts "I survived the drive up to VVR" if that's any indication to you of the conditions of the road. It can be done in just about any car, but be prepared for some interesting (and stunning) rough-road driving.

From Prather, take CA 168 north to the first stop sign. Turn left to stay on CA 168 past Shaver Lake and Sierra Summit Ski Resort. At Huntington Lake, turn right for Edison Lake and follow a good road for 6 miles. The next 14 miles are on an intimidating and winding one-lane road with potholes the size of small craters and lots of gravel. Allow at least two hours from this juncture. It appears as if they did not move a single boulder or tree in the creation of the road, thus it remains absolutely one lane the whole way, despite the fact that it takes traffic in both directions. Rest assured that there are pull-outs along the way. The first feat is going over Kaiser Pass (9,128 feet), then the road drops for close to 3,000 feet, only to climb close to another 2,000 feet back up to the lake level. It is not recommended to drive this road at night, and it's highly encouraged to have snow chains on hand year-round. A mile past the U.S. Forest Service High Sierra Ranger Station, take a left to head toward Edison Lake. Roll down and then up the mountain and follow a sign that reads "Vermilion Valley Resort 2 miles." Congratulations—you've arrived! And you thought the hard part was the hiking. . . .

GPS coordinates	*Starting trailhead* Red's Meadow Resort
UTM zone (WGS84)	11S
Easting	0316915
Northing	4165147
Latitude	N 37°36'51.37"
Longtitude:	W 119°04'30.50"

	Ending trailhead Lake Edison Ferry Landing
UTM zone (WGS84)	11S
Easting	0328251
Northing	4141859
Latitude	N 37°24'26.21"
Longitude	W 118°56'26.24"

4 Vermilion Valley Resort to Florence Lake

SCENERY: ✿ ✿ ✿ ✿	HIKING TIME: *2–5 days*
TRAIL CONDITION: ✿ ✿ ✿ ✿	OUTSTANDING FEATURES: *Bear Creek*
CHILDREN: ✿	*Meadow, Rosemarie Meadow, Marie Lake,*
DIFFICULTY: ✿ ✿ ✿ ✿	*Selden Pass, Sallie Keyes Lakes, Blayney Hot Springs*
SOLITUDE: ✿ ✿	*(optional)*
DISTANCE: *27 miles*	

This is a short route by John Muir Trail standards but a great stretch of the trail for hikers who want to be in more remote backcountry than a shorter trip normally affords. The short mileage allows you to carry more food, and it's possible to really stretch out this journey; lingering at stunning Marie Lake, leisurely ascending Selden Pass (10,880 feet), and allowing for a layover day at Sallie Keyes Lakes. It's also possible to make this section rather glamorous by spending the night at the Muir Trail Ranch or soaking in nearby Blayney Hot Springs. But this will depend on the ranch's availability for one-night stays, which can be quite limited. Admittedly the path begins with a grueling set of switchbacks shortly after the ferry from Edison Lake. Well-acclimated thruhikers will have little trouble, but anyone starting out from this point will get a rather rapid and heart-pounding introduction to the high-altitude hiking that awaits.

🚶🚶 After bidding good-bye to the home-cooked goodness and flushing toilets of Vermilion Valley Resort (VVR), climb onto the ferry for the 20-minute ride across Edison Lake and return to the backcountry. Ferries depart regularly during the hiking season (generally June 1 to October 1; seasonally dependent on snowpack) at 9 a.m. and 4 p.m., but private departures can be arranged for a fee. If you prefer to walk, it's 4.8 miles to return to the JMT from VVR along the northwestern shore of Edison Lake.

The ferry landing is changeable depending on weather and water conditions, so simply look for the trail heading northeastward up the valley. After 1.4 miles, you'll reach a sign for Selden Pass. Follow this trail across the bridge and continue your gentle uphill grade. About a

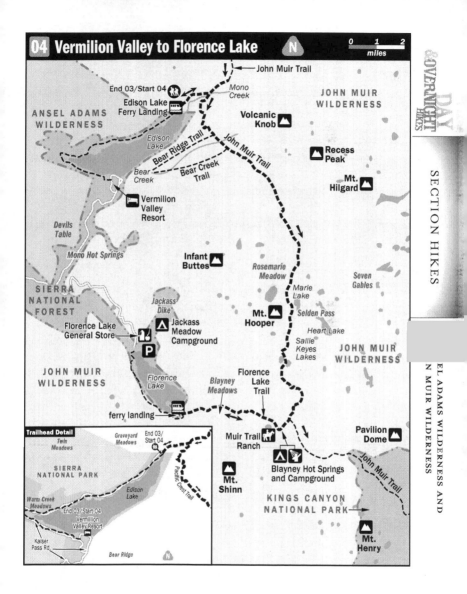

04 Vermilion Valley to Florence Lake

John Muir Trail

End 03/Start 04
Edison Lake
Ferry Landing

Mono
Creek

JOHN MUIR
WILDERNESS

ANSEL ADAMS
WILDERNESS

Volcanic
Knob

Edison
Lake

Bear Ridge Trail

John Muir Trail

Recess
Peak

Bear
Creek

Bear Creek
Trail

Mt.
Hilgard

Vermilion
Valley
Resort

Devils
Table

Mono Hot Springs

Infant
Buttes

Rosemarie
Meadow

Seven
Gables

SIERRA
NATIONAL
FOREST

Jackass
Dike

Marle
Lake

Florence Lake
General Store

Jackass
Meadow
Campground

Mt.
Hooper

Selden Pass

Heart Lake

Sallie
Keyes
Lakes

JOHN MUIR
WILDERNESS

P

JOHN MUIR
WILDERNESS

Florence
Lake

Blayney
Meadows

Florence
Lake
Trail

ferry landing

Pavilion
Dome

Trailhead Detail

Graveyard
Meadows

End 03/
Start 04

Muir Trail
Ranch

Twin
Meadows

SIERRA
NATIONAL PARK

Pacific Crest Trail

Edison
Lake

Mt.
Shinn

Blayney Hot Springs
and Campground

Warm Creek
Meadows

End 03/Start 04
Vermillion
Valley Resort

KINGS CANYON
NATIONAL PARK

John Muir Trail

Kaiser
Pass Rd

Bear Ridge

Mt.
Henry

half mile after crossing the bridge, traverse a stream from Mono Creek; a good place to top off water for the hot, dry climb that lies ahead. If you want to delay the climb, or if you got a late start, there is decent camping here.

The infamous switchbacks up to Bear Ridge begin here. The introduction is a gentle 15 switchbacks before the path levels out briefly through aspen groves. When the switchbacks continue, they are an unrelenting ascent of more than 2,000 feet. The trail is mostly shaded from the glare of the sun, but this doesn't stop it from being grueling. It's not that the grade is particularly steep, but most hikers have full bellies from VVR and packs heavy with newly refreshed food caches. Take it slowly. Reaching the top, the trail levels out to continue along Bear Ridge with excellent views south to Mount Hooper.

Descend slightly and ignore the Bear Ridge trailhead (9,835 feet) to the right, as this would bring you back to VVR in 5.7 miles. Descend through aspen groves, fording the creek many times, and soak in the gorgeous open views and vibrant wildflowers in this section. The scenery changes as the sky opens up between the conifers to views of the mountains. Wildflower buffs will go wild for the brilliant display of Indian paintbrush, Yosemite aster, shooting stars, and mariposa lilies. There is plenty of cow parsnip, a favorite among

ELEVATION PROFILE

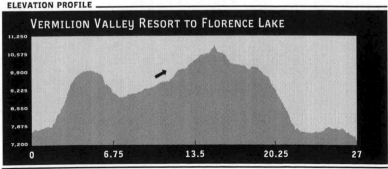

VERMILION VALLEY RESORT TO FLORENCE LAKE

bears, as the trail descends via switchbacks through alternating thickets of pine forest, aspen, and manzanita.

Reach another junction, this time with the Bear Creek trailhead, but continue straight, climbing up-canyon along lovely Bear Creek. There is excellent camping, swimming, picnicking, and feet-soaking opportunities along the banks of the creek. Travel on a nice gentle path, ignoring the turnoff for Seven Gables Lake, and cross Hilgard Creek, which can be difficult in early season. Gradually ascend 500 feet toward Upper Bear Creek Meadow (9,575 feet), an area that can be buggy in July and August.

Switchback steeply up 500 feet to reach Rosemarie Meadow, and junctions to Sandpiper, Lou Beverly, and Rose lakes. The camping is excellent here. Just past the Rose Lake junction (10,030 feet), cross the West Fork Bear Creek and continue rising another 500 feet to Marie Lake (10,551 feet). Marie sits like a sapphire set in granite snow-covered mountains. Here, as in other Sierra locations, the snow often takes on a pinkish hue. This "watermelon snow" phenomenon is the result of an algae bloom. And while it smells sweet, it would be truly regrettable to eat it. This is another excellent place to camp, albeit rather exposed. Continue rising on steep switchbacks, rocky and exposed, above Marie Lake to Selden Pass (10,900 feet). Get your windbreaker out and savor the views for as long as you can.

Wind down a moderate grade to romantically shaped Heart Lake, rife with swimming, fishing, and napping opportunities. It's common to see quite a few day-trippers traveling on horseback from the Muir Trail Ranch here. Continue gently descending past Sallie Keyes Lakes' glacial blue waters ringed with trees. Traverse through the middle of the two sister lakes on a flat and beautiful walk that provides respite from the day's formidable climbing and descending. There is plenty of great camping here amid the trees. The lakes are named for the daughter of one of the original Diamond D Ranch (now Muir Trail Ranch) owners, a nearby rural guesthouse that has been privately owned since 1885.

There is one last climb on a hot and exposed rise after a meadow, followed by a descent through alternating sunlit meadows, switchbacks, and aspen groves over the next 5 miles. A series of loose dirt and exposed rock switchbacks winds down into the river canyon through low-lying manzanita shrubs. Often horse trains pass, and there is evidence of their presence on the trail as well. Watch your step!

Arrive at a junction at 8,380 feet. The southeast path continues on the JMT toward Kings Canyon National Park, but we follow the southwest path to the Florence Lake Trail and the Muir Trail Ranch. Veering right, continue descending along dusty, steep switchbacks giving way to even more arduous ones upon nearing the Muir Trail Ranch. Reach a second junction within less than a mile with trails that head northwest to Florence Lake or southwest toward the Muir Trail Ranch.

If you are packing out at Florence Lake, turn right to hike the 4.5 miles to the ferry landing (7,350 feet). The trail to Florence Lake can be a bit confusing, as numerous pack trails intersect it. Continue heading downhill through lodgepole forests and meadows, with the San Joaquin River on your left (albeit not always visible) and success will certainly come. There is a rough gravel jeep road used by the Muir Trail Ranch that carries supplies from the ferry to the ranch that frequently intersects the trail.

From late May until late September, the ferry runs every day, weather permitting. From the trail, there are scheduled departures to the Florence Lake Store at 9 and 11 a.m. and 1, 3, and 5 p.m. Unless you have a very large group of people (30 or more), reservations are not necessary. Use the radiotelephone at the landing to call the store, and they will send a boat at the next scheduled time. You can purchase your ticket (one-way adults, $10; children ages 12 and under, $5) when you arrive.

For Muir Trail Ranch (MTR), continue straight and stay right at the Y intersection to pick up food caches or spend the night in a cabin (reservations required). Descend past the junction and enter through the gate next to the horse corral. Turn right through a second metal gate and ring the hiker's tin can bell for assistance. While certainly helpful, the MTR does not afford nearly the warm reception of Vermilion Valley Resort. They will happily store your food caches (a whopping $45 to send it here), but they aren't too interested in hikers in any other capacity. You can't eat here, their hot springs are for guests only, and there's no camping. That being said, they have a great storage house of food that other hikers have abandoned, and they will gladly let you forage for extra trail mix. They are open to receiving hikers during daylight hours. (See page 21 for more information on sending food.)

Established in the 1800s, the ranch was here well before the John Muir Trail was completed in 1947, and it occupies close to 200 acres straddling the river. For the most part, MTR caters to its own clientele of weeklong stays, where guests eat at the ranch and take day excursions to nearby lakes and valleys on horseback. Recently, they have launched a "shorter stay" program that allows hikers to stay overnight for one night and use all their amenities. It's worth contacting them well in advance if you'd like to take advantage of this and join the ranks of Clark Gable and Carole Lombard, who slumbered here in the 1940s. Normally they have more availability for one-night stays in the shoulder season. See Directions following for contact information.

To camp nearby, return to the last junction and follow signs to Blayney Hot Springs. It can be crowded here, and the hot springs aren't incredibly self-evident. Ford the river (difficult when full) and walk to the far end of the meadow to a series of somewhat muddy pools with wooden logs around the perimeter. The water is about chest high on an adult, and there's room for close to eight people in the largest spring. It's usually too hot in the day to enjoy the springs, but they are wonderful at night. Keep in mind, however, that you need to ford the river again after enjoying your steamy dip.

PERMIT INFORMATION: *Permits that originate in the Sierra National Forest can be reserved by mail only. Applications can be mailed to High Sierra Ranger District, Attention: Wilderness Permits, P.O. Box 559, Prather, CA 93651. You can call*

(559) 855-5360 for questions, but you cannot reserve a permit over the phone. Year-round office hours are 8 a.m. to 4:30 p.m. daily. You may download a wilderness-permit application at **www.fs.fed.us/r5/sierra/passes/getwild permit.shtml**. Or you may include the following in your written request: name; address; daytime phone number; number of people in the party; method of travel (foot); number of stock (if applicable); start and end dates; proposed camping areas for each night; entry and exit trailheads (Lake Edison entry, Florence Lake exit); principal destination; money order or check (made out to the U.S. Forest Service) for a nonrefundable $5-per-person processing fee. No credit cards are accepted.

You can pick up your permit at the High Sierra Ranger District, en route to Edison and Florence lakes. The station can be found on Kaiser Pass Road (Forest Service Road 80), off CA 168 coming from Prather.

About 60 percent of permits are reservable, while the remainder are set aside as walk-in permits. You can get a walk-in permit at the High Sierra Ranger District as well.

DIRECTIONS: VERMILION VALLEY RESORT—To get to Vermilion Valley Resort (VVR), you will most likely need a friend to pick you up or try your hand at hitchhiking. The closest main highway is CA 168, 30 miles northeast of Fresno, but the final 14 to 20 miles of your journey is a feat to be applauded. VVR even makes a T-shirt that boasts "I survived the drive up to VVR," if that's any indication to you of the road conditions. It can be done in just about any car, but be prepared for some interesting (and stunning) rough-road driving.

From Prather, take CA 168 north to the first stop sign. Turn left to stay on CA 168 past Shaver Lake and Sierra Summit Ski Resort. At Huntington Lake, turn right for Edison Lake and follow a good road for 6 miles. The next 14 miles are on an intimidating and winding one-lane road with potholes the size of small craters and lots of gravel. Allow at least two hours from this juncture. It appears as if they did not move a single boulder or tree in the creation of the road, thus it remains absolutely one lane the whole way, despite the fact that it takes traffic in both directions. Rest assured that there are pull-outs along the way. The first feat is going over Kaiser Pass (9,128 feet), then the road drops for close to 3,000 feet, only to climb close to another 2,000 feet back up to the lake level. It is not recommended to drive this road at night, and it's highly encouraged to have snow chains on hand year-round. A mile past the U.S. Forest Service High Sierra Ranger Station, take a left to head toward Edison Lake. Roll down and then up the mountain and follow a sign that reads "Vermilion Valley Resort 2 miles." Congratulations—you've arrived! And you thought the hard part was the hiking. . . .

FLORENCE LAKE—The trail ends at the ferry landing for Florence Lake. The drive here is almost identical to the drive to VVR (above), but when you reach the U.S. Forest Service High Sierra Ranger Station, take a right to head toward Florence Lake (instead of the left to reach Edison Lake). Drive the remaining 6.5 miles to Florence Lake Resort, which offers a store and ferry service across the lake. Buy your ferry ticket here, then move your car to long-term parking in the paved lot above the store. If you choose to walk instead, add an additional 4 miles to your journey along the western shore of the lake.

MUIR TRAIL RANCH—To make reservations at Muir Trail Ranch for a shorter stay, call (209) 966-3195, fax (209) 966-7895, visit www.muirtrailranch.com, or e-mail howdy@muirtrailranch.com. An overnight stay in their tent or log cabins ranges from $125 to $150, including breakfast, a sack lunch for the trail, and dinner. If horses are available, it may be possible to arrange transport from the ranch to the ferry landing at Florence Lake. It's $200 to transfer luggage via packhorse and an additional $50 if you'd like to ride a horse yourself.

GPS Trailhead Coordinates	*Starting trailhead* LAKE EDISON FERRY LANDING
UTM zone (WGS84)	11S
Easting	0328251
Northing	4141859
Latitude	N 37°24'26.21"
Longitude	W 118°56'26.24"

GPS Trailhead Coordinates	*Ending trailhead* FLORENCE LAKE FERRY LANDING
UTM zone (WGS84)	11S
Easting	0327479
Northing	4123903
Latitude	N 37°14'41.32"
Longitude	W 118°56'46.47"

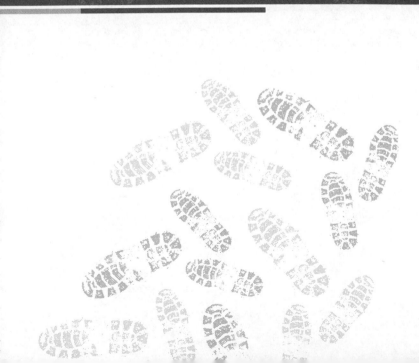

John Muir Wilderness;
Kings Canyon and
Sequoia National Parks

FLORENCE LAKE,
ROADS END, ONION VALLEY,
MOUNT WHITNEY

In the high altitude, you soar above the treeline with wide granite expanses and endless views. In lower elevations, relish the rich diversity of flora in sunny meadows and shady forest thickets. Throughout, find a range of lakes, streams, rivers, and distinct ecosystems

5 Florence Lake to South Lake

SCENERY: ✪ ✪ ✪ ✪ ✪	DISTANCE: 45 miles
TRAIL CONDITION: ✪ ✪ ✪ ✪	HIKING TIME: 5–7 days
CHILDREN: ✪	OUTSTANDING FEATURES: Blayney
DIFFICULTY: ✪ ✪ ✪ ✪ ✪	Hot Springs, Evolution Valley, Muir Pass,
SOLITUDE: ✪ ✪ ✪	Le Conte Canyon, Dusy Basin, Bishop Pass

Arguably one of the most beautiful and challenging stretches along both the John Muir and Pacific Crest trails, this section traverses the renowned Evolution Valley, a remote high–altitude wonderland of jagged peaks, glacial cirques, stark alpine lakes, and wildflower–strewn meadows. And the remote locale, combined with some difficult climbs, nearly ensures some degree of solitude. It's possible to begin your journey with a soak in nearby hot springs before you rise through Evolution Valley and the lofty heights of Muir Pass (11,955 feet) in the heart of Sequoia and Kings Canyon national parks. After dropping down into Le Conte Canyon, your journey leaves the JMT to venture east through the sparse forest and granite bowls of Dusy Basin and up to amazing Bishop Pass (11,972 feet). Descending toward Owens Valley, enjoy the region's many high–altitude lakes and meadows.

🚶 Packs (and hopefully bellies!) full, climb onto the water taxi for the 20-minute ride across Florence Lake. From late May until late September, the ferry runs every day, weather permitting. There are scheduled departures to the trailhead at the eastern end of the lake at 8:30 and 10:30 a.m. and 12:30 , 2:30, and 4:30 p.m. Unless you have a very large group of people (30 or more), reservations are not necessary. If you prefer to walk, add an additional 4 miles to your journey along the western shore of the lake.

Begin the steep uphill walk over slabs of Sierra granite. After 0.5 miles, bear left to distance yourself from Florence Lake Road, a Jeep service road that serves the Muir Trail Ranch and frequently inter-sects the trail. The route from Florence Lake can be a bit confusing, as numerous pack trails intersect it. Simply remember to continue

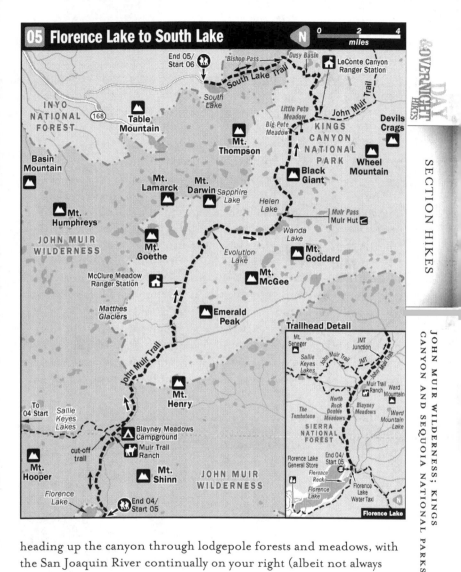

05 Florence Lake to South Lake

N

0   2   4
miles

End 05/
Start 06

Bishop Pass

Dusy Basin

LeConte Canyon
Ranger Station

South Lake Trail

John Muir Trail

INYO
NATIONAL
FOREST

168

South
Lake

Little Pete
Meadow

Table
Mountain

KINGS

Big Pete
Meadow

CANYON

Devils
Crags

Mt.
Thompson

NATIONAL

PARK

Wheel
Mountain

Basin
Mountain

Mt.
Lamarck

Mt.
Darwin

Sapphire
Lake

Black
Giant

Mt.
Humphreys

Helen
Lake

Muir Pass
Muir Hut

JOHN MUIR
WILDERNESS

Mt.
Goethe

Evolution
Lake

Wanda
Lake

Mt.
Goddard

McClure Meadow
Ranger Station

Mt.
McGee

Matthes
Glaciers

Emerald
Peak

Trailhead Detail

Mt.
Seneger

JMT
Junction

John Muir Trail

John Muir Trail

JMT

Muir Trail
Ranch

Ward
Mountain

To
04 Start

Sallie
Keyes
Lakes

Mt.
Henry

North
Rock
Double
Meadows

Blayney
Meadows

Ward
Mountain
Lake

The
Tombstone

Blayney Meadows
Campground

SIERRA

Muir Trail
Ranch

NATIONAL

cut-off
trail

FOREST

Mt.
Hooper

Mt.
Shinn

JOHN MUIR

Florence Lake
General Store

End 04/
Start 05

WILDERNESS

Florence
Rock

Florence
Lake

End 04/
Start 05

Florence
Lake

Florence
Lake
Water Taxi

Florence Lake

heading up the canyon through lodgepole forests and meadows, with
the San Joaquin River continually on your right (albeit not always
visible) and success will certainly come. After another 2 miles, ford

Alder Creek and travel through Blayney Meadows. Within one more mile, reach the western boundary gate of the Muir Trail Ranch.

Unless you have reservations or are picking up food caches, the Muir Trail Ranch (MTR) is not open to the public. A private establishment since the 1800s, the ranch was here well before the John Muir Trail's completion in 1947, and it occupies close to 200 acres straddling the river. Originally called the Diamond D ranch, its name was changed in later years to reflect proximity to the trail, and they have been providing food cache services to hikers for well over 50 years. For the most part, MTR caters to its own clientele of week-long stays, where guests eat at the ranch and take day excursions to nearby lakes and valleys on horseback. Recently, they have launched a "shorter stay" program that allows hikers to stay overnight for one night and use all their amenities. It's worth contacting them well in advance if you'd like to take advantage of this. Normally, they have more availability for one-night stays in the shoulder season. See Directions following for contact information.

Walk about 1 mile through the ranch, following the barbed-wire fence line, before reaching the eastern boundary gate. To camp and soak in the public hot spring nearby, bear right (south) on the first spur trail beyond the gate to Blayney Hot Springs. The camping can be quite

ELEVATION PROFILE

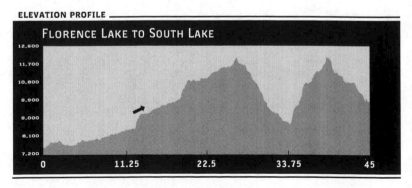

FLORENCE LAKE TO SOUTH LAKE

crowded here, and the hot springs aren't incredibly self-evident. Ford the river (difficult when full) and walk to the far end of the meadow to a series of somewhat muddy pools with wooden logs around the perimeter. The water is about chest high on an adult, and there's room for close to eight people in the largest spring. It's usually too hot in the day to enjoy them, but they are wonderful at night. Keep in mind, however, that you need to ford the river again after enjoying your steamy dip.

If you have the energy and aren't in the mood for a soak, there is better camping if you walk a mile and half past Blayney Hot Springs to wide-open campsites right by the river. Bears are bold in this area, no-doubt sensing fresh food in hiker's packs. Do not sleep with food in your tent!

Within moments of passing the spur trail, pass another junction indicating the John Muir Trail (JMT) to the right (north). Ignore this, and continue rising moderately over another 1.5 miles through the densely wooded San Joaquin Canyon to another junction where the JMT will once again join our path. Stay right and continue traveling southeast toward Kings Canyon and Piute Pass on the main trail. At the end of small rise, come into an open view of the San Joaquin River on the right.

Disregard the Piute Trail to your left and cross a steel bridge over Piute Creek to leave John Muir Wilderness and enter Kings Canyon National Park, following signs to Evolution Valley. Continue hiking along the South Fork San Joaquin River through alternating stands of quaking aspen groves and exposed granite and rock. Nice campsites dot the way amid thickets of Jeffrey Pine, sage, and chaparral. Continue across a red steel bridge and past more campsites winding gently up-canyon through forest and meadow. Meander through wildflowers and shady woods, gradually rising along this gentle path until you reach Franklin Meadow (8,480 feet) and a trail junction with the path to Goddard Canyon. Turn left to cross the bridge over the river. There are numerous campsites on both sides of the river if you want to call it a day.

Head northward briefly before beginning a series of steep, exposed rocky stairs. One mile and 500 feet of climbing after the junction, listen for the thundering cascades of Evolution Creek as it tumbles down the staircases of rock. It's an experience usually heard before seen. The grade of the ascent wanes here as the trail follows closely next to the roaring creek hurtling its way downstream. There are plenty of opportunities for a good foot soaking on the water-strewn granite rocks, but use caution in the swift current. There is camping along the river here, and the cool breeze of the water brings the temperature down several degrees. Continue ascending this lush riverside paradise colored with wildflowers.

Ford the swift-moving Evolution Creek—often a shoes-off affair even later in the season—and pass through Evolution Meadow. This area is deadly with bugs in the middle of summer, but provides decent camping in the shoulder season. Continue climbing moderately to McClure Meadow and its seasonally staffed ranger station (9,660 feet). There are numerous excellent campsites here, one tucked closely behind the ranger station as well as several along the meadow. It's advised to walk away from the water a bit to find less buggy sites if the mosquitoes are out in full force.

From the meadow, walk a gentle grade for 1.5 miles to neighboring Colby Meadow (9,840 feet). About 2 miles past McClure Meadow, there are a number of Darwin Creek crossings, which can be difficult during high water amid downed logs. Find more campsites after the crossings. Break out into a more open granite area before heading back into the trees to begin your ascent to Evolution Lake. After crossing the 10,000-foot marker, the climb stiffens to steep switchbacks. Happily, much of the trail is coolly shaded for the beginning of the climb. Coming out of the trees, continue on exposed rock switchbacks that will lead to Evolution Lake. Gorgeous and stark, this is the beginning of one of the most spectacular stretches of the hike through a barren region carved by ice some 10,000 years ago. Before reaching the lake, cross a flowered meadow and enjoy the initial stunning views. Evolution Lake (10,850 feet) is desolate and rocky but boasts a colorful display of fiery shooting stars and eye-catching tiger lilies along its creek. There is limited camping among clusters of white-bark pines on the lake's northern shore.

The naming of Evolution Lake is a bit of a California phenomenon, where instead of famed leaders or religious figures, scientists, geneticists, and evolutionists are honored. Most of the names in this region are thanks to Theodore S. Solomons, an early explorer, photographer, and writer. Often called the "Pioneer of the John Muir Trail," Solomons was one of the first to traverse Evolution Valley in 1895 and is credited with accurately surveying and mapping this stretch of Sierra topography. His maps were instrumental in the trail's creation.

Enjoy a bit of respite as the trail flattens out on a moderate to gentle ascent toward Sapphire Lake. Look for streaming waterfalls and wily marmots en route to the second set of climbs. Cross over the river on an impressive path of well-placed large stepping stones. Skirt Sapphire Lake, truly the color of its name, and begin a series of switchbacks gaining altitude again along the hulking side of Mount Huxley. The trail levels as you come up to an unnamed lake before the final climb up and over to Wanda Lake (11,426 feet), so named for John Muir's eldest daughter. There is little to no camping here, and the gnats are annoyingly friendly. Follow the northeast shore of this deceptively long lake (stretching more than a mile) and begin a rocky 2.2-mile ascent up the barren granite-strewn country that lies ahead.

From here, look for the Muir hut at the top of the pass in the distance on a rocky saddle in the Goddard Divide. Muir Pass is the only Sierra pass to boast a man-made structure. The stone hut, built by the Sierra Club in 1931, is intended as a refuge for hikers in inclement weather. The fireplace is stoned-in, but the unlocked emergency shelter still offers protection from wind, ice, and rain. Be watchful of marauding mice ever hopeful for a dropped peanut, however!

The hut comes in and out of view as you switchback up various rises. Dwarfed by neighboring peaks of Mount Warlow and Mount Goddard, the pass shouldn't appear too high or intimidating, and indeed the initial ascent is rather gradual through the stone rubble. The trail turns into a stony walkway with occasional rough-hewn stairs. Cross the outlet to Lake McDermand, usually made easy by a stepping-stone bridge, and continue up the rocky switchbacks to Muir Pass (11,955 feet). Camping is forbidden on the ridge, as there's no place to dispose of human waste.

After savoring the view, descend on rocky zigzags toward an unnamed glacial snowmelt lake. Continue switchbacking down, sometimes over snowfields in early season, dropping a little more than a mile to stunning Helen Lake (11,617 feet), named for Muir's second daughter. There is limited exposed camping here. Cross the outlet of Helen Lake, a difficult feat when the water's high, and conquer another obstacle course crossing the southern side of a small marshy tarn.

Drop down into meadow and continue lowering toward treeline, hugging the canyon wall along the Middle Fork Kings River. As you lose elevation, the landscape becomes more lush and green as the river navigates its way down the valley. Riverside campsites can be found beyond Helen Lake by climbing up some of the ridges along the trail. Water is fairly omnipresent. Continue the stunning descent into the valley past wildflowers, snowmelt streaming down the canyon wall, and unnamed lakes with gorgeous greenish hues reflecting the trees. The trail, choked with manzanita, narrows as you descend. At times, it's rocky and steep, but it gradually gives way to wood thickets and meadow.

Arrive at Big Pete Meadow (9,200 feet) followed by an aspen grove and, in another mile, Little Pete Meadow (8,880 feet). Ironically, the second meadow is the larger of the two, but there is lots of good riverside camping in both of these areas. Meander through a section of lovely ferns descending farther into Le Conte Canyon. There is a ranger station (8,750 feet; manned from June to mid-September) near the junction with the trail to Dusy Basin.

There are lovely wooded campsites along the river just below the ranger station.

Hikers continuing on the JMT would head straight southward following the Middle Fork Kings River. Instead, turn left to leave the JMT and begin the steep eastward ascent of more than 3,000 feet toward Bishop Pass. Embark on the first of two sets of switchbacks through a swath of forest along the Dusy Branch of the Kings River. The second set heads through the sparsely forested Dusy Basin. For camping, pass north of the lowest lake and ascend a side trail to campsites at the largest northernmost lake nearly 5 miles from the trail junction.

From the main trail, follow the sandy path up the final eastward pitch to Bishop Pass (11,972 feet) and enjoy northern views of the Inconsolable Range and the arid Owens Valley in the distance. Descend neatly through stunted white-bark pines (and sometimes through snowfields) toward Bishop Lake, and follow the east shore of Saddlerock Lake (11,128 feet), 2 miles below the pass. Cross the lake's outlet on a footbridge and enjoy a moderate descent through rocky tundra past Timberline Tarns, a chain of small glacially carved lakelets. Traverse high above Spearhead Lake, and cross above Ruwau Lake's outlet on a stepping-stone path. Ignore the side trail to Ruwau Lake and continue to the southern end of Long Lake, nestled beneath Chocolate Peak, where high-altitude campsites may be found (10,753 feet). Enjoy spectacular views southward to Mount Goode. It is a mere 2 miles to the trailhead from here.

Ignore the side trails to Bull and Chocolate lakes and continue zigzagging down the rocky trail toward the timberline. Ignore the trail to Mary Louise Lakes on your right, and shortly thereafter, traverse a lovely meadow crossing the lake's outlet on a small footbridge. Just past this junction, the Treasure Lakes Trail joins from the left to continue its northern journey through lodgepole pines and fir trees. Admire northeastern views of towering Hurd Peak. Ascend briefly and then continue downhill, exiting the wilderness on two small footbridges above the east side of South Lake (9,768 feet).

PERMIT INFORMATION: *Permits that originate in the Sierra National Forest can be reserved by mail only. Applications can be mailed to High Sierra Ranger District, Attn: Wilderness Permits, P.O. Box 559, Prather, CA 93651. You can call (559) 855-5360 for questions, but you cannot reserve a permit over the phone. Year-round office hours are 8 a.m. until 4:30 p.m. daily. You may download a wilderness-permit application at www.fs.fed.us/r5/sierra/passes/getwildpermit.shtml. Or you may include the following in your written request: name; address; daytime phone number; number of people in the party; method of travel (foot); number of stock (if applicable); start and end dates; proposed camping areas for each night; entry and exit trailheads (Lake Edison entry, Florence Lake exit); principal destination; money order or check (made out to the U.S. Forest Service) for a nonrefundable $5-per-person processing fee. No credit cards are accepted.*

You can pick up your permit at the High Sierra Ranger District, en route to Edison and Florence lakes. The station can be found on Kaiser Pass Road (Forest Service Road 80), off CA 168 coming from Prather.

About 60 percent of permits are reservable, the remainder are set aside for walk-in permits. You can get a walk-in permit at the High Sierra Ranger District as well.

DIRECTIONS: FLORENCE LAKE TRAILHEAD—The trail begins at the ferry landing for Florence Lake. To get to Florence Lake you will most likely need a friend to pick you up or try your hand at hitch-hiking. The closest main highway is CA 168, 30 miles northeast of Fresno, but the final 20 miles of your journey is a feat to be applauded. It can be done in just about any car, but be prepared for some interesting (and stunning) rough-road driving.

From Prather, take CA 168 north to the first stop sign. Turn left to stay on CA 168 past Shaver Lake and Sierra Summit Ski Resort. At Huntington Lake, turn right for Edison Lake and follow a good road for 6 miles. The next 14 miles are on an intimidating and winding one-lane road with potholes the size of small craters and lots of gravel. Allow at least two hours from this juncture. It appears as if they did not move a single boulder or tree in the creation of the road, thus it remains absolutely one lane the whole way, despite the fact that it takes traffic in both directions. Rest assured that there are pull-outs along the way. The first feat is going over Kaiser Pass (9,128 feet), then the road drops for close to 3,000 feet, only to climb close to another 2,000 feet back up to the lake level. It is not recommended to drive this road at night, and it's highly encouraged to have snow chains on hand year-round. A mile past the U.S. Forest Service High Sierra Ranger Station, take a right to head toward Florence Lake (instead of the left to reach Edison Lake). Drive the remaining 6.5 miles to Florence Lake Resort, which offers a store and ferry service across the lake. You can buy your ferry ticket here (one-way adults, $10; children ages 12 and under, $5), but then you need to move your car to long-term parking about a quarter mile back form the store on Florence Lake Road. Congratulations—you've arrived! And you thought the hard part was the hiking. . . .

Taking public transit to Florence Lake is near impossible and would require hitchhiking at some point along the way.

MUIR TRAIL RANCH—To make reservations at Muir Trail Ranch for a shorter stay, call (209) 966-3195, fax (209) 966-7895, visit www.muirtrailranch.com, or e-mail howdy@muirtrailranch.com. An overnight stay in their tent or log cabins ranges from $125 to $150, including breakfast, a sack lunch for the trail, and dinner. If horses are available, it may be possible to arrange transport from the ranch to the ferry landing at Florence Lake. It's $200 to transfer luggage via packhorse and an additional $50 if you'd like to ride a horse yourself.

SOUTH LAKE TRAILHEAD—The closest town to the South Lake trailhead is Bishop, on US 395, 39 miles southeast of Mammoth Lakes and 15 miles north of Big Pine. From Bishop, drive west 15 miles on CA 168 (West Line Street) to the South Lake Road junction. Turn left and travel 7 miles to the Bishop Pass trailhead and parking. Overnight parking is found on the upper lot.

You can take public transit as far as Bishop via Inyo Mono Transit's CREST bus, but you will need to walk or hitchhike the remaining 22 miles to the trailhead. The bus travels north on US 395 between Bishop and Reno via Mammoth Lakes on Tuesday, Thursday, and Friday, and south between Mammoth Lakes and Ridgecrest on Monday, Wednesday, and Friday. There is also limited Saturday service between Bishop and Mammoth Lakes only. For Mammoth Lakes transit info, please see directions for Tuolumne to Red's Meadow (page 75). Rates and routes are subject to frequent change; call ahead for information and reservations at (760) 872-1901 or (800) 922-1930. More information can be found on the Web at www.countyof inyo.org/transit/CRESTpage.htm.

Lastly, you could contact the friendly folks at Mammoth Shuttle by phone at (760) 934-6588 to arrange for private transit on demand to or from the trailhead. This is a pricey option but may be worth it for larger groups. Prices range considerably from $100 (from one eastern-Sierra trailhead to another) to $600 (from Mammoth to Kings Canyon). The price to go from Mammoth to Yosemite averages $200 (per eight-passenger shuttle, not per person).

GPS coordinates	*Starting trailhead* FLORENCE LAKE FERRY LANDING
UTM zone (WGS84):	11S
Easting	0327479
Northing	4123903
Latitude	N 37°14'41.32"
Longitude	W 118°56'46.47"

GPS Trailhead Coordinates	*Ending trailhead* SOUTH LAKE
UTM zone (WGS84):	11S
Easting	0361118
Northing	4115144
Latitude	N 37°10'20.67"
Longitude	W 118°33'51.77"

6 South Lake to Roads End
in Kings Canyon National Park

SCENERY: ✩ ✩ ✩ ✩	HIKING TIME: *6–8 days*
TRAIL CONDITION: ✩ ✩ ✩ ✩	OUTSTANDING FEATURES: *Bishop Pass,*
CHILDREN: ✩	*Dusy Basin, Le Conte Canyon, Golden Staircase,*
DIFFICULTY: ✩ ✩ ✩ ✩	*Palisade Lakes, Mather Pass, Lake Marjorie,*
SOLITUDE: ✩	*Pinchot Pass, Castle Domes, Mist Falls*
DISTANCE: *58 miles*	

This east-to-west section is laden with high-altitude passes for hungry peak-baggers. With alpine lakes, craggy peaks, and flower-strewn meadows rewarding considerable effort, this is high drama, Kings Canyon—style. The journey begins at an already formidable altitude, so rugged above-treeline views are within grasp almost immediately. Crest Bishop Pass (11,972 feet) and soak in the silent grandeur of the peaks of the Inconsolable Range. Summit Mather Pass (12,100 feet) via cleverly camouflaged switchbacks up a seeming pile of rubble, and finally reach the highest prize of the section: Pinchot Pass (12,130 feet) where the thin air does not spoil a rich view. A long descent past meadows, aspen groves, and thundering waterfalls leads to end of the road at the namesake canyon of Kings Canyon National Park.

🏃 From the parking lot, follow a rocky trail on the east side of South Lake (9,768 feet) and cross two small footbridges. Descend briefly and then begin climbing through lodgepole pines and fir trees with Hurd Peak looming to the south. Bishop Pass, the first of three high-altitude passes in this journey, waits patiently a little more than 5 miles and 2,000 feet ahead.

Continue through intermittent aspen groves and after less than a mile, bear left away from the Treasure Lakes Trail to continue ascending southeast. After another half mile, ignore the Marie Louise Lakes Trail and bear right to travel south. Repeat this pattern with the Bull Lake Trail shortly thereafter. After 2 miles and 900 feet

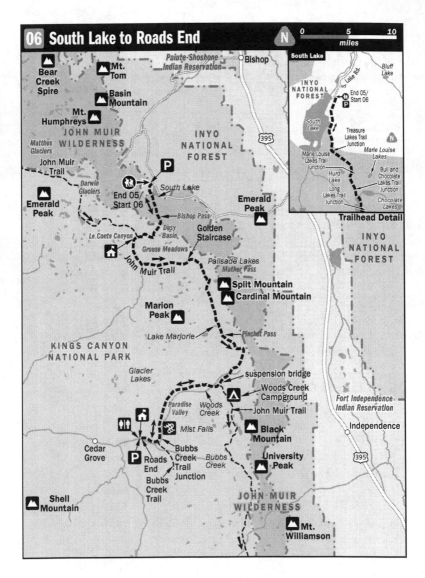

0   5   10
miles

N

South Lake

Bishop

Paiute-Shoshone
Indian Reservation

Bear
Creek
Spire

Mt.
Tom

Basin
Mountain

Mt.
Humphreys

**JOHN MUIR
WILDERNESS**

Matthes
Glaciers

John Muir
Trail

Darwin
Glaciers

**INYO

NATIONAL

FOREST**

395

Trailhead Detail

**INYO
NATIONAL
FOREST**

St. Lake Rd.

End 05/
Start 06

Bluff
Lake

South
Lake

Treasure
Lakes Trail
Junction

Marie Louise
Lakes

Marie Louise
Lakes Trail
Junction

Hurd
Lake

Bull and
Chocolate
Lakes Trail
Junction

Long
Lakes Trail
Junction

Chocolate
Lakes

Emerald
Peak

End 05
Start 06

South Lake

Bishop Pass

Dusy
Basin

**Golden
Staircase**

Emerald
Peak

Le Conte Canyon

Grouse Meadows

John Muir Trail

Palisade Lakes

Mather Pass

Split Mountain

Cardinal Mountain

**INYO

NATIONAL

FOREST**

**Marion
Peak**

Lake Marjorie

Pinchot Pass

**KINGS CANYON
NATIONAL PARK**

Glacier
Lakes

suspension bridge

Woods Creek
Campground

Paradise
Valley

Woods
Creek

John Muir Trail

Mist Falls

**Black
Mountain**

Fort Independence
Indian Reservation

Independence

Cedar
Grove

Roads
End

Bubbs
Creek
Trail
Junction

Bubbs
Creek

Bubbs
Creek

**University
Peak**

395

Bubbs
Creek
Trail

**Shell
Mountain**

**JOHN MUIR
WILDERNESS**

**Mt.
Williamson**

of climbing from the trailhead, reach the southern end of Long Lake, nestled beneath Chocolate Peak, where high-altitude campsites may be found (10,753 feet). Enjoy spectacular views southward to Mount Goode. Despite the relatively low mileage, it's wise to acclimate to the altitude before pushing onward.

Follow the eastern shore of Long Lake, ignoring the side trail to Ruwau Lake, and bear right to continue a southward ascent through rocky tundra past Timberline Tarns, a chain of small glacially carved lakelets. Enjoy northeastern views of towering Hurd Peak upon reaching Saddlerock Lake (11,128 feet), and cross its outlet on a footbridge. From here, it's a 2-mile push, some of it seemingly near vertical, through stunted white-bark pines and the occasional snowfield to Bishop Pass (11,972 feet), resting high above Bishop Lake. Enjoy backward northern views of the Inconsolable Range and the arid Owens Valley, while ahead lie the plunging canyons of Kings Canyon National Park.

Leaving John Muir Wilderness, descend into Kings Canyon along a sandy granite trail westward toward lake-filled Dusy Basin. Le Conte Canyon lies some 6 miles, and more than 3,000 feet, below. The first campsites are about a mile below the pass on a side trail toward the largest northernmost lake. From the main trail, descend

ELEVATION PROFILE

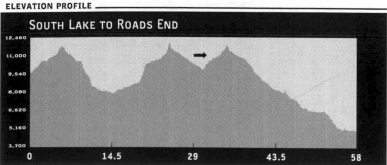

steeply down two sets of switchbacks through the sparse forest, several river crossings, and a lovely hanging valley to the junction with the John Muir Trail (JMT). A ranger station (8,750 feet; manned from June to mid-September) sits just west of this trail crossing, and there are lovely wooded campsites along the river just below the station.

From this junction, turn left to descend southward on the JMT following the Middle Fork Kings River. Shortly after the ranger station, cross a wooden and steel footbridge over Dusy Branch and continue descending through alternating aspen groves and wood thickets. Manzanita encroaches on the narrow trail, so long pants are advised for this section. Arrive at grassy Grouse Meadows, where camping is good and plentiful as long as the area is not closed for restoration, as it is occasionally. Three miles from the ranger station, come to a junction with the trail to Roads End (8,070 feet). Ignore this and turn left to follow the JMT east up a small rise and continue climbing gently toward Deer Meadow. It's advised, however, to pump water before beginning this dry 800-foot climb.

Cross a verdant pasture of long grasses and traverse a sandy rise through sweet-smelling sage bushes and horsetail ferns to reach Deer Meadow, thick with lodgepole pines. Campsites begin appearing at the northern end of the meadow and continue along its length. In the buggy season, Deer Meadow can feel like a dark and murky swamp, and it's best to wait until the trail rises almost to the end of the meadow for more-open sites with better access to water and fire pits. This is the last place to camp before climbing up to the Palisade Lakes, so bear this in mind before forging ahead.

Leaving Deer Meadow, ford Glacier Creek and begin the climb of the famed Golden Staircase, an ascent of 1,700 feet over 3 miles with no accessible campsites. As climbs go, it's incredibly well graded, and the consistent pitch allows for a certain rhythm in your hiking. In fact, it's impossible not to appreciate the beauty of this engineering feat that allows you (hopefully) to maintain a sense of humor while ascending Mather Pass. At times it seems impossible to determine how the trail will wind its way up the steep granite peaks surrounding you. Interestingly, these granite cut stairs were the last leg of the JMT to be completed. Fantastic views back toward the valley provide the perfect excuse for a break to breathe in the fragrant sage. Currants and wildflowers line the staircase in a pleasantly distracting manner as well. Ascend the first 1,000 feet in less than a mile and a half up carefully carved switchbacks. Try to climb early or in the late afternoon before intense sun bakes the stone.

As the switchbacks lessen, come to a meadow surrounded by the soaring peaks of the Palisades Group, where Lower Palisade Lake (10,613 feet) hides behind a low rise. Surrounded by a cirque, the lake is deep and beautiful, but doesn't offer much in the way of camping on the windy ridge. Skirt the lake briefly before beginning another rocky, switchbacked climb. As you gain altitude, Upper Palisade Lake (10,679 feet) reveals herself on the rise, less than 100 feet higher than her sister lake. The trail doesn't actually descend to the lake, but there is nice protected camping amid the dwarfed white-bark pines, and plentiful water from Palisade Creek.

Continue rising and traverse a stream at 11,200 feet. This is a good place to stop for water and sunscreen, as the next leg consists of dry, exposed, rocky switchbacks. The landscape is a barren one of granite shards and a few snowmelt tarns. Be sure to savor views back toward Palisade Lakes. It's difficult to see the path ahead as it switchbacks smoothly up and back: an optical illusion of boulder-sized granite chunks. At times the trail travels over fist-sized rocks and other times more finely crushed pebbles. Named for the first head of the National Park Service, Stephen Mather would have enjoyed the endless views from his beautiful, silent, and stark namesake pass (12,100 feet).

Descend sharply along zigzagged switchbacks to desolate Upper Basin. After a mile or so, the grade eases and it's a moderate 5-mile descent past glittering tarns to treeline. The desert rockscape, with the stately presence of aptly named Cardinal Mountain, eventually gives way to lush woodland as it parallels the South Fork Kings River.

As the river bends southwest, the trail heads southeast on the trail. Use caution in this river crossing. There are good campsites on both sides of the river with rotating areas closed for restoration.

After the river crossing, the trail gently rises and fords the creek again (difficult in early spring). Begin ascending more steeply via pine-shaded switchbacks where there is no camping available. At the junction with the Taboose Pass Trail, continue straight while the grade eases up, and enter a bucolic open meadow. After a quarter mile, reach another junction with trails leading northeast to Taboose Pass and southwest to Bench Lake. Ignore these and continue walking up the peaceful valley, keeping the river on your left. There is excellent camping among these mountain tarns and grassy meadowland.

Keep ascending past multiple lakelets, including bluer-than-blue Lake Marjorie (11,132 feet), whose sparkling deep recesses lie ringed by a cirque on one side and by trees on the other. Climb away from Marjorie on steep switchbacks. The lake on the shelf above Marjorie is a pure turquoise to Marjorie's electric azure.

Unlike Mather and Muir, the approach to Pinchot Pass is less of a clear switchback to the top, and there are many deceptively false summits as the trail winds briefly north before the final ascent. Follow a series of shale zigzags up to the col sitting between eastern Mount Wynne and western Crater Mountain, admiring the fireweed tucked into unlikely crevices. When finally reached, the colors of Pinchot Pass (12,130 feet) are arresting: bright yellow-green lichen stands out on the gray rock, while the mountains ahead are a tempered warm rust color.

Descend steep serpentine loose rock switchbacks. As the grade lessens, enjoy a rolling downhill through a landscape of dwarfed and stunted trees searching for proper nutrients in the reddish soil. Glittering alpine lakes nestle in the arms of towering granite peaks, providing excellent camping with a view.

The switchbacks steepen once again shortly before passing the junction with the Sawmill Pass Trail (10,346 feet). Good campsites can be found along Woods Creek. Here, the descent becomes gentler again, following the river on a high ridgeline as the trail sinks farther into the lush canyon.of the

Near the confluence of Woods Creek and the South Fork Kings River, reach a junction with the trail to Roads End. Veer right to leave the JMT, which continues on a dramatic suspension bridge over Woods Creek to an established campsite with bear boxes. Instead continue a gradual rollicking descent with the grand towers of Castle Domes on the right and Woods Creek on the left.

The trail continues rolling downward through the narrow canyon walls. Intermittent campsites are easily found amid the meadows and aspen groves, although it's a bit of a struggle to get to the water due to streamside shrubs. Cross the South Fork Kings River on an impressively robust stone-and-steel bridge built in 2006 to reach the campsites of Upper Paradise Valley (6,876 feet), where camping is restricted to one night in designated spots in an effort to help this fragile area recover from frequent use. There are bear boxes, a pit toilet, and numbered sites at each Paradise Valley campground (lower, middle, and upper). Drop another 2.2 miles through blackberry bushes and open meadow to Middle Paradise Valley (6,619 feet), where sugar and ponderosa pines provide shade and there's a sandy riverside beach. Travel a final 1.1 miles downhill through ferns and forest to Lower Paradise Valley (6,586 feet). The streamside campsites on the left are the nicest in terms of shade and proximity to water. Bear sightings are frequent here.

Leaving Lower Paradise Valley, the trail becomes steeper and rockier along the river. The descent to Mist Falls (5,563 feet) is an excruciating series of granite stairs that mock tired knees. The reward is a magnificent display of thundering cataracts and cooling mist, as per the waterfall's name. Continue down and turn right at the junction with the Bubb's Creek Trail. From here, it's a flat 2-mile walk to the trailhead, but the wide sandy road can be scorching on a summer day as it absorbs and reflects the heat. Cross Copper Creek on a small footbridge to reach the parking lot and ranger station at Roads End (5,036 feet). At the parking lot there are decadently luxurious amenities such as a bathroom with a pit toilet, toilet paper (usually), a water spigot, some picnic tables, garbage-disposal cans, and bear boxes. Ah, civilization.

PERMIT INFORMATION: *Permits that originate in the Inyo National Forest can be reserved by contacting the Wilderness Permit Reservation Office (351 Pacu Lane, Suite 200, Bishop, CA 93514). They are open 8 a.m. to 4:30 p.m. daily from June 1 to October 1, and Monday through Friday during the rest of the year. You can reserve over the phone at (760) 873-2483, by fax at (760) 873-2484, or by mail. You will need to provide the following information: name; address; daytime phone number; number of people in the party; method of travel (foot); number of stock (if applicable); start and end dates; entry and exit trailheads (South Lake entry, Roads End exit); principal destination; credit-card number and expiration date, money order, or check for a nonrefundable $5-per-person processing fee.*

You can then pick up your permit at the White Mountain Ranger Station (798 North Main Street, Bishop, CA 93514). Office hours are 8 a.m. to 5 p.m.; (760) 873-2500. About 60 percent of permits are reservable; the remainder are set aside for walk-in permits.

DIRECTIONS: SOUTH LAKE TRAILHEAD—The closest town to the South Lake trailhead is Bishop, on US 395, 39 miles southeast of Mammoth Lakes and 15 miles north of Big Pine. From Bishop, drive west 15 miles on CA 168 (West Line Street) to the South Lake Road junction. Turn left and travel 7 miles to the Bishop Pass trailhead and parking. Overnight parking is found in the upper lot.

You can take public transit as far as Bishop via Inyo Mono Transit's CREST bus, but you will need to walk or hitchhike the remaining 22 miles to the trailhead. The bus travels north on US 395 between Bishop and Reno via Mammoth Lakes on Tuesday, Thursday, and Friday, and south between Mammoth Lakes and Ridgecrest on Monday, Wednesday, and Friday. There is also limited Saturday service between Bishop and Mammoth Lakes only. For Mammoth Lakes transit info, please see directions for Tuolumne Meadows to Red's

Meadow. Rates and routes are subject to frequent change; call ahead for information and reservations at (760) 872-1901 or (800) 922-1930. More information can be found on the Web at www.county ofinyo.org/transit/CRESTpage.htm.

Lastly, you could contact the friendly folks at Mammoth Shuttle by phone at (760) 934-6588 to arrange for private transit on demand to or from the trailhead. This is a pricey option but may be worth it for larger groups. Prices range considerably from $100 (from one eastern-Sierra trailhead to another) to $600 (from Mammoth to Kings Canyon). The price to go from Mammoth to Yosemite averages $200 (per eight-passenger shuttle, not per person).

ROADS END TRAILHEAD—Roads End lies at the head of the canyon for which the park is named. From Fresno, head 53 miles east on CA 180 to Kings Canyon's Big Stump Entrance, continue straight through the park, dropping more than 3,000 feet as the road curves along the South Fork of the Kings River to Grant Grove Village. It's another 30 miles to Cedar Grove Village, and Roads End lies another 6 miles east at its terminus.

Public transit is sorely lacking in the park. Your best bet would likely be to hitchhike to Fresno (serviced by Amtrak and Greyhound) or to contact Mammoth Shuttle for a trailhead-to-trailhead ride (see above).

GPS coordinates	*Starting trailhead* SOUTH LAKE
UTM zone (WGS84):	11S
Easting	0361118
Northing	4115144
Latitude	N 37°10'20.67"
Longitude	W 118°33'51.77"

GPS Trailhead Coordinates	*Ending trailhead* ROADS END
UTM zone (WGS84):	11S
Easting	0358790
Northing	4073406
Latitude	N 36°47'40.82"
Longitude	W 118°35'4.16"

7 Roads End *to Onion Valley*

SCENERY: ✿ ✿ ✿ ✿ ✿	DISTANCE: *35 miles*
TRAIL CONDITION: ✿ ✿ ✿ ✿	HIKING TIME: *4–5 days*
CHILDREN: ✿	OUTSTANDING FEATURES: *Mist Falls, Paradise*
DIFFICULTY: ✿ ✿ ✿ ✿	*Valley, Rae Lakes, Glen Pass, Kearsarge Pass*
SOLITUDE: ✿	

Much of this section mirrors the venerable Rae Lakes Loop, one of Kings Canyon's most celebrated hikes. Its popularity is not surprising given that it squeezes nearly every alpine highlight into a jam-packed 35-mile adventure: waterfalls, wood thickets, riverside valleys, picturesque alpine lakes, high-mountain passes, and stunning views of jagged peaks. Starting with a moderate climb, rise through lush Paradise Valley before joining the John Muir Trail as it crosses Woods Creek on a spectacular suspension bridge. Continue ascending up-canyon to reach the justifiably famed Rae Lakes, a chain of gorgeous high-altitude lakes sitting below Glen Pass (11,978 feet). If time allows, plan a layover day at Rae Lakes to loll about in supreme alpine splendor before summiting the pass. Descending toward Vidette Meadow, continue south while the Rae Lakes Loop returns west to the trailhead. Leaving the JMT, head east rising to yet another lofty perch at Kearsarge Pass (11,845 feet) before exiting the wilderness in Onion Valley.

𝕏 From Roads End trailhead (5,036 feet), follow the Paradise Valley Trail. Just past the ranger station, cross Copper Creek on a footbridge and continue east. It's a flat 2 miles on exposed pumice sand from the ranger station to the junction with Bubbs Creek Trail. Walk through fragrant stands of pine and cedar that ultimately give way to a shaded fern grove. At the Bubbs Creek junction, veer left uphill for the moderate 2.7-mile journey up to Mist Falls (5,563 feet). Head north along the South Fork Kings River through open forest and along granite staircases. The dramatic views down the valley provide plenty of excuses to stop and catch your breath. Reach Mist Falls, so called for the glistening spray erupting from its base,

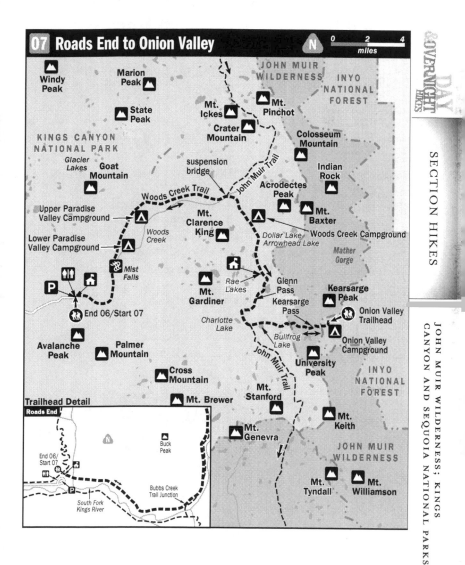

Windy Peak

Marion Peak

State Peak

Mt. Ickes

Mt. Pinchot

JOHN MUIR WILDERNESS

INYO NATIONAL FOREST

Crater Mountain

Colosseum Mountain

KINGS CANYON NATIONAL PARK

Glacier Lakes

Goat Mountain

suspension bridge

John Muir Trail

Indian Rock

Acrodectes Peak

Woods Creek Trail

Upper Paradise Valley Campground

Mt. Clarence King

Mt. Baxter

Woods Creek

Woods Creek Campground

Dollar Lake Arrowhead Lake

Lower Paradise Valley Campground

Mather Gorge

Mist Falls

P

Rae Lakes

Mt. Gardiner

Glenn Pass

Kearsarge Peak

Kearsarge Pass

Onion Valley Trailhead

End 06/Start 07

Charlotte Lake

Bullfrog Lake

Onion Valley Campground

Avalanche Peak

Palmer Mountain

John Muir Trail

University Peak

INYO NATIONAL FOREST

Cross Mountain

Mt. Brewer

Mt. Stanford

Mt. Keith

Trailhead Detail

Roads End

Buck Peak

Mt. Genevra

JOHN MUIR WILDERNESS

End 06/Start 07

P

Bubbs Creek Trail Junction

South Fork Kings River

Mt. Tyndall

Mt. Williamson

JOHN MUIR WILDERNESS

and admire one of Kings Canyon's largest waterfalls. This is a popular destination for day hikers and families. After reaching the thundering falls, the real climbing begins. Head up a series of tight switchbacks through a landscape of cottonwoods and aspen groves for 2 miles to Lower Paradise Valley.

Once you reach Paradise Valley, camping is restricted to one night in designated spots in an effort to help this fragile area recover from frequent use. There are bear boxes, a pit toilet, and numbered sites at each Paradise Valley campground (lower, middle, and upper). The streamside sites at Lower Paradise Valley (6,586 feet) are some of the nicest in terms of shade and proximity to water. Hikers aren't the only people who love this trail; it's also a mecca for savvy bears looking to pick up a little extra trail mix. Be sure to store your food well.

Continue up-valley another 1.1 miles to Middle Paradise Valley (6,619 feet), where sugar pines and butterscotch-scented ponderosa pines shade sites and a sandy riverside beach affords excellent views. It's another 2.2 miles along the river to Upper Paradise Valley (6,876 feet). Walk through the well-defined campsite and cross the South Fork Kings River on an impressively robust stone-and-steel bridge built in 2006. This marks the confluence of Woods Creek and the

ELEVATION PROFILE

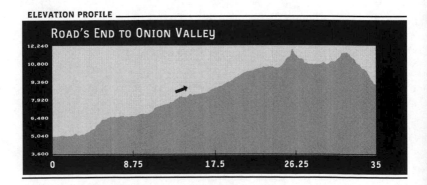

ROAD'S END TO ONION VALLEY

132

South Fork Kings River. Head east along the Woods Creek Trail, ascending up the wooded valley.

Descend to Castle Dome Meadow, an area strewn with aspen groves and boasting stunning afternoon light. Designated campsites are no longer necessary past Paradise Valley. There are places to camp on the west side of the meadow, although it's a bit of a struggle to get to the water due to streamside shrubs. It's not a struggle, however, to crane your neck to enjoy views of the highly polished summits of Castle Dome's royal peaks. And it's a treat to dry your clothes on the omnipresent sage bushes that impart a lovely scent. Nature's deodorant!

Leaving the meadow, continue eastward, reentering the forest, and continue to climb intermittent steps carved into the tough granite. Descend among cottonwoods and enter a grove of older aspen trees just before the trail meets the John Muir Trail (JMT), coming down from Pinchot Pass.

Interestingly, quaking aspen are the most widely distributed tree in the northern hemisphere. While celebrated for their flat leaves that shimmer in the wind and provide a brilliant fall display, they are most unique for their reproductive cloning. Each aspen grove lives off a single root system, where new trees, "suckers," are sent up when older trees are destroyed. The width of the tree trunk indicates the age of that particular tree, but some of the groves themselves are 8,000 years old. Their regeneration tactics make aspens often the first species to grow in a zone following a disturbance, such as a fire or avalanche.

Turn right to follow the JMT south across the impressively sound and robust suspension bridge. Built in 1988, this is the mack daddy of bridges, certain to withstand whatever Woods Creek sends its way. Late in the season, when the creek is but a trickle, it seems a tad over-wrought, but its girth and weight are a welcome find during high water. Be sure to cross one person at a time.

Across the bridge, note the popular Woods Creek campsites

(8,492 feet) scattered amid Jeffrey Pines with bear boxes. This is an excellent place to pump water. Ignore the side trails to western campsites and continue heading southeastward on the Rae Lakes Loop. The trail begins rising gently and subsequently switchbacking up through an open area of aspen trees. The landscape alternates between rocky switchbacks and more open valleys and meadows along this gradual ascent.

Cottonwoods give way to lodgepole pines as the trail winds its way into a fragile meadow near the Baxter Creek crossing. This is another excellent spot for water, as the climb up to Dollar Lake is a hot and dry one. Continue climbing as the trail rises above the river. The views open up tremendously above treeline. Walk past foxtail pines to Dollar Lake (10,200 feet) for your first taste of the alpine wonderland that awaits at Rae Lakes. There is limited camping here, but check signs for restoration areas.

Skirt the lake's western shore and continue climbing to larger Arrowhead Lake (10,300 feet), nestled under the impressive Fin Dome peak, a sharklike protrusion reflected in the placid waters. Campsites dot the northeast lakeshore.

Cross Arrowhead's outlet and walk along the lake's eastern shore until the trail begins climbing again, away from the water. Reach the first lake in the Rae Lakes chain, with campsites with bear boxes near the south end. Just past this first lake, a spur trail veers right to the seasonally staffed Rae Lakes Ranger Station (10,597 feet). The lakes were named by William Colby, a Sierra Club member instrumental in the founding of Kings Canyon National Park, who honored his wife, Rachel ("Rae").

Campsites are plentiful here, as are jaw-dropping views, and this is an excellent place for a layover day or two. There is a two-night camping limit at each Rae Lake. Follow the trail southwest for close to a mile across a flat isthmus dividing Middle and Upper Rae lakes and admire the photogenic granite islands "floating" in the upper lake.

From here, it's a 2-mile grunt up nearly 1,500 feet to the top of Glen Pass, and you should get water before starting the climb. Ignore the rough trail heading northwest toward Sixty Lake Basin, and continue south toward the pass.

Mount an initial set of steep switchbacks before the trail levels out briefly to follow a surprising lush brook among willows into a meadow swale worthy of an Andy Goldsworthy project.

A second set of switchbacks leads to a more desolate landscape of turquoise tarns and rocky ridgelines. There is little vegetation here, save for the occasional stunted white-bark pine. Limited camping is available here if you're willing to sleep on a granite bed.

Continue on a final series of gratifying zigzags up the talus slope to the narrow ridge of Glen Pass (11,978 feet). Admire southwestern views of snow-covered Mount Brewer and the reddish slopes of Mount Bago, as well as other Great Western Divide peaks.

Descend serpentine switchbacks past an unnamed lake. The descending trail can be hard to pinpoint amid snow and scree, but look for helpful cairns and continue heading southwest. Eventually the switchbacks become more defined. Head down gravelly angled paths toward treeline and a number of lovely tarns, an excellent place to fill up on water. Continue down, bump up a small rise, then enjoy a long, gradual descent along the ridgeline above Charlotte Lake as white-bark and foxtail pines come into view. Admire views of looming Charlotte Dome hovering above the distant lake. Descend into an open wash with lots of junctions. Hikers continuing to Mount Whitney would continue straight, ignoring the side trails to Kearsarge Pass and Bullfrog Lake over the next mile.

Instead, veer left at the first junction following Glen Pass to leave the JMT and head east toward Kearsarge Pass. Traverse a rocky slope high above Bullfrog and Kearsarge lakes to ascend the 2.7 miles to Kearsarge Pass (11,823 feet). Catch your breath and admire epic views of Kearsarge Pinnacles and Lakes. Descend east a grueling

5 miles, with close to 3,000 feet of elevation loss, to the Onion Valley Trailhead (9,180 feet).

PERMIT INFORMATION: *Reservations are available in Kings Canyon National Park from May 21 through September 21. Mail or fax your application to Wilderness Permit Reservations, Sequoia and Kings Canyon National Parks, 47050 Generals Highway, #60, Three Rivers, CA 93271. For more information, call (559) 565-3708. Applications can be downloaded at* **www.nps.gov/seki/planyourvisit/ wilderness_permits.htm,** *or you can furnish the following information with your written request: name; address; daytime phone number; number of people in the party; method of travel (foot); number of stock (if applicable); start and end dates; proposed camping areas for each night; entry and exit trailheads (Roads End entry, Whitney Portal exit); principal destination; credit-card number and expiration date, money order, or check made out to the National Park Service for a nonrefundable $15 reservation fee.*

You may pick up your permit beginning at 1 p.m. the afternoon preceding the beginning of the hike, and it will be held until 9 a.m. the morning of the hike. If you know you will be delayed, call the Roads End Ranger Station, (559) 565-3766 to hold your reserved permit. But note that they cannot hold your permit past 2:30 p.m., as the station closes at that time. Walk-in permits are also available at the Roads End Ranger Station, however this is a busy trailhead and walk-in permits are sometimes limited.

DIRECTIONS: ROADS END TRAILHEAD—Roads End lies at the head of the canyon for which the park is named. From Fresno, head 53 miles east on CA 180 to Kings Canyon's Big Stump Entrance, continue straight through the park, dropping more than 3,000 feet as the road curves along the South Fork Kings River to Grant Grove Village. It's another 30 miles to Cedar Grove Village, and Roads End lies another 6 miles east at its terminus.

Public transit is sorely lacking in the park, and your best bet would be to hitchhike from Fresno (serviced by Amtrak and Greyhound) or to contact the friendly folks at Mammoth Shuttle by phone at (760) 934-6588 to arrange for private transit on demand to or from the trailhead. This is a pricey option but may be worth it for larger groups. Prices (per eight-passenger shuttle, not per person) range considerably from $100 (from one eastern-Sierra trailhead to another) to $600 (from eastern- to western-Sierra trailheads).

ONION VALLEY TRAILHEAD—The closest town to the Onion Valley trailhead is Independence on US 395, 16 miles north of Lone Pine and 26 miles south of Big Pine. From Independence, drive west on Market Street for 13 miles. The road name eventually changes to Onion Valley Road, and the trailhead lies at its terminus (9,180 feet).

You can take public transit as far as Independence via Inyo Mono Transit's CREST bus, but you would need to walk or hitchhike the remaining 13 miles to the trailhead. The bus travels north on US 395 between Bishop and Reno via Mammoth Lakes on Tuesday, Thursday, and Friday, and south between Mammoth Lakes and Ridgecrest on Monday, Wednesday, and Friday. Independence lies 45 minutes south of Bishop. Rates and routes are subject to frequent change; call ahead for information and reservations at (760) 872-1901 or (800) 922-1930. More information can be found on the Web at www.countyofinyo.org/transit/CRESTpage.htm.

GPS coordinates	*Starting trailhead* ROADS END
UTM zone (WGS84):	11S
Easting	0358790
Northing	4073406
Latitude	N 36°47'40.82"
Longitude	W 118°35'4.16"

GPS Trailhead Coordinates	*Ending trailhead* ONION VALLEY
UTM zone (WGS84):	11S
Easting	0380432
Northing	4070625
Latitude	N 36°46'25.95"
Longitude	W 118°20'23.37"

8 Onion Valley to Mount Whitney

SCENERY: ✿ ✿ ✿ ✿ ✿	DISTANCE: *51 miles*
TRAIL CONDITION: ✿ ✿ ✿ ✿	HIKING TIME: *5–7 days*
CHILDREN: ✿	OUTSTANDING FEATURES: *Gilbert Lake,*
DIFFICULTY: ✿ ✿ ✿ ✿ ✿	*Kearsarge Pass, Vidette Meadow, Forester Pass,*
SOLITUDE: ✿	*Guitar Lake, Mount Whitney.*

The final section of the John Muir Trail is not for the weak of heart, literally or figuratively. With two significant mountain passes to climb, and the conquering of the contiguous United State's highest peak thrown in, this is where hikers earn their bragging rights. However, this 51-mile journey is not just for peak-bagging glory hounds; it also includes some of the most spectacular alpine scenery that the Sierras have to offer. Those who love their vistas wide can have their fill of expansive hiking above treeline—open meadows, stark lakes, and the cold embrace of ringing mountains nearly everywhere. Begin with a hefty 2,600-foot climb up to Kearsarge Pass (11,823 feet), where the trail descends to Vidette Meadow before it's time to hoof it up foreboding Forester Pass (13,120 feet). Catch your breath descending to Tyndall Creek before another scenic traverse up to Guitar Lake. Lastly, conquer the inimitable Mount Whitney, a giant granite dome hulking over the Owens Valley. Like a benevolent mother, she lures the minions to join her in the heavens. That is, until you get halfway up and she begins to feel like a deceptively wicked and cruel illusionist, ever farther away. Until, finally, you reach the seeming top of the world.

🚶🚶 The trail from Onion Valley starts off with a bang, with a nearly 12,000-foot pass found less than 6 miles from the start. However, the trailhead (9,185 feet) begins at such a high altitude that it's not quite as daunting as one may fear. Begin climbing a series of manzanita-choked switchbacks to a wooded thicket. Follow babbling Independence Creek up 700 feet to Little Pothole Lake (9,900 feet). Stop and rest under the shade of willow trees before tackling the next set of switchbacks to Gilbert Lake. Traverse the lake's northern shore on a more gradual ascent to the northern shore of shallow

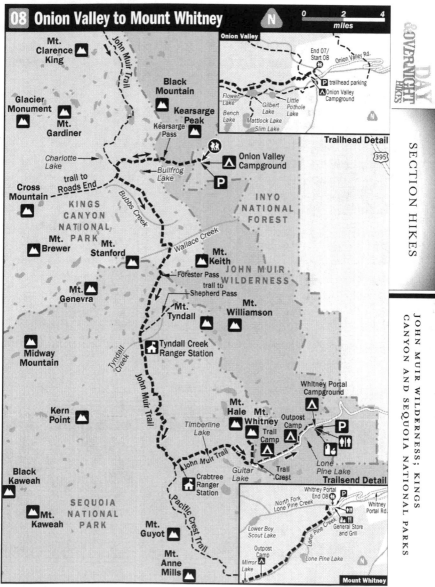

Flower Lake. Once again begin ascending a series of rocky switch-backs, first past lovely Heart Lake, then above the granite wall that hides Big Pothole Lake. From here, sweat up two final switchbacks to Kearsarge Pass (11,823 feet). Catch your breath and admire epic views of Kearsarge Pinnacles and Lakes.

Begin descending on a narrow, rocky trail. At the first junction, veer left to travel south on a spur trail toward Bullfrog Lake. Camp-sites lie 1 mile below the pass at Kearsarge Lakes (10,960 feet). Skirt the lakes' northern shores to continue a moderate descent west toward Bullfrog Lake (10,610 feet), another reliable water source. At the next junction, turn left to join the southern route of the John Muir Trail (JMT).

Continue descending in the canyon, crossing Bullfrog Lake's outlet, and arrive at lower Vidette Meadow (9,550 feet). Ignore the trail to Roads End, and head southeast on the JMT toward Forester Pass and upper Vidette Meadow. Enjoy a level path along the river through the shady woods of Vidette Meadow (9,600 feet), passing numerous campsites with bear boxes, before beginning a gradual to moderate forested ascent along Bubbs Creek.

Ignore the unmarked spur trail heading east to Center Basin, and continue southeast, passing more campsites, to ford Center Basin

ELEVATION PROFILE

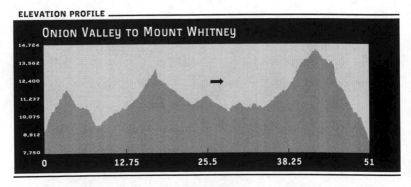

ONION VALLEY TO MOUNT WHITNEY

Creek. Rising out of the valley on rocky switchbacks, the view opens up tremendously en route to Forester Pass. Hitting the 11,000-foot mark, enjoy a gradual plateau with magnificent views of the snowy spires and sheer granite cliffs surrounding the rocky rubble.

Continue climbing up nicely graded switchbacks, as a stream tumbles over small boulders and tundralike grass. Just above 12,000 feet there is a glittering tarn below the distinctive jagged spire of Junction Peak. From here, continue ascending the impressive stone bridge notched into the side of the mountain supporting the trail. There is little apparent life this high, but it's possible to spot the occasional bird, marmot, and renegade wild currants thriving in the thin air. The route winds beneath a ridgeline (don't be deceived that this is the pass!) before ending with a series of tight, steep switchbacks to a narrow windswept niche.

Forester Pass (13,120 feet) straddles the boundary between Kings Canyon and Sequoia national parks. Officially, Forester Pass is considered the highest pass on the JMT. This is because the summit of Mount Whitney, the trail's technical terminus, is not a pass. However, these are just technicalities, because you must traverse Trail Crest (13,656 feet) to descend to Whitney Portal. However, by all accounts, Forester is an impressively high perch from which to admire the sweeping views below.

Descend on one of the most cleverly engineered paths of the JMT. Twisty curves bend and wrap around near-impossible geography to create grades that even sore knees can appreciate. Wind down this structurally incredible labyrinth of serpentine switchbacks until they gradually give way to fast walking on a moderate descent toward the timberline. Pass gorgeous tarns and boulder fields with plenty of accessible water.

Just past the junction for Lake South America, descend again and arrive at bear boxes and campsites that boast stunning sunset alpenglow on the western mountains next to rushing Tyndall Creek (10,890 feet). After fording the river, pass the trail to the Tyndall

Creek Ranger Station, and shortly thereafter come to a spur trail leading to Shepherd Pass. Ignore this and follow the first signpost to Mount Whitney, 16.1 miles ahead. Begin a short but steep climb. Cross the outlet to Tyndall Frog Ponds to find more tent sites and a bear box. Continue up- and downhill through shade and open ridge, gradually rising into Bighorn Plateau. Enjoy epic views of Tawny Point to the east and a desolate lake on your left. Remember this lake, as it's possible to view it from the final stretch of trail toward Mount Whitney. Begin descending again through woodland toward Wallace Creek.

Cross Wright Creek and continue rising and descending toward Wallace Creek and the junction with the High Sierra Trail (10,405 feet). Use caution fording Wallace Creek. There are bear boxes and campsites on the right. Ascend 500 feet through forested benches, until the trail levels out at Sandy Meadow. Continue a pleasantly flattish route along a forested ridge before climbing over a ridge and dropping down through wooded thicket to the junction with a trail to Crabtree Meadow (10,880 feet). This is where the Pacific Crest Trail (PCT) and JMT part ways for the final time. The PCT continues heading south toward its terminus in Mexico, while the JMT turns left to head east toward Mount Whitney.

After a little less than a mile through shady conifers, come to a second junction (10,640 feet) with a trail to nearby Crabtree Ranger Station. At the signpost, look for a plastic bin with waste-disposal "pack it out" kits for those continuing to Guitar Lake and the Whitney Zone. These glamorous "wag bags" come with toilet paper, hand sanitizer, and deodorant gel. In recent years the composting toilets en route from Whitney Portal cannot keep up with the number of hikers. In 2006, more than 30,000 people camped in the Whitney Zone. As a result, the forest service is asking all backpackers to pick up the provided wag bags and pack out *all* their trash. There are disposal bins at Whitney Portal upon arrival at the trailhead.

Wag bag securely stashed, climb gradually for 1.5 miles to photogenic Timberline Lake (11,070 feet), where Mount Whitney's southwestern flank is reflected in her glassy waters, making even amateur photographers feel like Ansel Adams. There is no camping at this lake.

Walk the lake's northern shore to begin the final climb up to Guitar Lake. The climb is a bit deceiving, seemingly always on the next rocky bench, despite being less than 2 miles from Timberline Lake. Traverse a lovely alpine meadow while mountains rise up to embrace you as you head skyward. You can't actually see Mount Whitney from Guitar Lake (11,450 feet). Camping is forbidden in the grassy areas of the lake, but there are several campsites around the neck of the guitar. Simply follow the use trail southwest for these tent sites with outstanding sunset views. Beware the hungry and clever marmot, as you will undoubtedly want food on your journey up Whitney!

Ascend to the next bench, passing the mirror ponds above Guitar Lake with limited camping. This is the last spot to pump water before the summit. Begin switchbacking up the west side of Whitney, huffing and puffing the nearly 2 miles from Guitar Lake to Trail Junction (13,484 feet), where the eastern trail from Whitney Portal meets the JMT. Foot traffic increases here as hordes of day hikers, in varying degrees of fitness and distress, summit Mount Whitney as well.

A handful of waterless campsites can be found just northwest of Trail Junction. Look for a small use trail leading to small tent sites surrounded by small rocks that create a wind shelter. While dry (and high!) these campsites are one of the world's best spots for sunset photography, and they provide an excellent point from which to get an early start on the summit. Many hikers rise and start walking in the dark to enjoy sunrise on the summit.

If you're not camping here, this is still the best place to shed your pack and lighten your load for the final climb. Be sure, however, not to leave any food that invites marauding animals to chew through your pack. While it's just shy of 2 miles to the top, with only about 1,000 feet of climbing at a moderate to gentle grade, the thin air makes the journey quite taxing. Be sure to bring food, water, and extra layers. And, of course, your camera!

Begin walking the rocky ridgeline, enjoying westward views to Mounts Hale and Young and beyond, and the pointed spire of Mount Muir to the east. Look for the unnamed lake in Bighorn Plateau that you passed nearly 12 miles ago. Rocky spires and narrow ledges provide endless photo opportunities. The climb can be a bit vertigo-inducing for some, so take it easy and admire the jagged landscape of stony outcroppings, narrow windows with views to Owens Valley, and asymmetrical rocks balanced in a seemingly precarious fashion on impossible ledges.

Round the corner around Keeler Needle, and begin the final ascent to the top of Mount Whitney (14,497 feet). Approaching the summit's broad plateau, it can be easy to lose the trail among the rocks. Watch for cairns until the tin-roofed shelter at the top comes into view. The shelter is a welcome spot during high winds, but do not seek protection here during a storm, as the tin roof is a lightning conductor. Hikers have died here in the past.

For JMT thru-hikers, this marks the completion of their task, as oddly enough the top of Whitney also marks the official end of the John Muir Trail. Even purists, however, manage to descend the trail eventually.

The mountain was christened Whitney in 1864 to honor Josiah Whitney, one of the chief surveyors of California and the author of a travel guide to Yosemite published in 1869. Whitney was a known advocate for creating a national park to protect Yosemite. Ironically, Whitney and John Muir engaged in a public battle as to the evolutionary origins of Yosemite Valley. Whitney scoffed at Muir's theory of glacial activity and derided Muir for being an uneducated sheepherder. Ironic, considering scientific data now supports Muir's hypothesis. And more ironic still that the bookend to the trail honoring John Muir is named after one of his rivals.

Either way, there's a palpable sense of victorious accomplishment in the air from all who reach the summit. There's a book to sign, housed in a steel box outside the shelter, that reveals the international flavor of all those who climb to Whitney's top. There is also a USGS survey marker to the east of the shelter among the big boulder rocks.

Flanked by neighboring 14,000 footers, Mounts Muir and Russell, Mount Whitney is a benign ruler towering above the Owens Valley. To the east, enjoy views of the Inyo Mountains and the Alabama Hills. To the south, Mount Hitchcock and Mount Langley greet the eye. To the west, admire the Sawtooth Peak, Kaweah Peaks, and the Great Western Divide. To the north lie Junction Peak, Mount Tyndall, and Mount Williamson, which just barely missed being the highest peak in the lower 48.

Keep your celebration in check, however, because it's important to conserve some energy for the descent. It's recommended that you leave the summit no later than 3 p.m., returning the way you came to Trail Junction. From here, turn left to hump over one more short but steep hill about 150 feet to Trail Crest (13,650 feet). Somehow knowing that this is the last climb makes it rather manageable. Enjoy views eastward to Owens Valley, your eventual destination. Descending from Trail Crest, you leave Sequoia National Park and fittingly reenter John Muir Wilderness. From here, it's truly all downhill. The descent begins with a tight set of steep switchbacks dynamited into the eastern side of the mountain. Cables provide assistance over an icy section about a mile from Trail Crest.

Trail Camp (12,000 feet) is the first legal camping area on the eastern side of the summit and lies more than 1,500 feet below Whitney. It is not without charm and enjoys lovely sunsets over a small tarn; however it's a far cry from the remote wilderness experienced to date. Often overcrowded with inexperienced backpackers, it can feel a bit like a garbage dump at times. There are solar toilets on the southern side of camp, but in recent years the toilets have not been able to keep up with the number of hikers, and they are often full toward the end of the season. It is for this reason that wag bags are being encouraged more and more. While it's less than ideal to have to pack your wag bag with you, you can rest easy in the knowledge that you're aiding environmental progress.

From Trail Camp, descend steep concrete stairs and reach a more gentle grade with several dry but flat campsites lining the route. Enjoy views of Consultation Lake in the distance to the south. Reach Mirror Lake (10,650 feet) after a little more than 2 miles of descent from Trail Camp. You cannot camp here, but it's a lovely spot to have a snack and gaze at the reflective water. Further down, pass Outpost Camp (10,367 feet) with its solar toilets and usually over-crowded tent sites. Continue traveling northeast and pass a spur trail to Lone Pine Lake (9,980 feet) to the right. If planning to camp again, it's worth it to make this slight detour to sleep by Lone Pine Lake, where dawn sunlight is to be appreciated.

Continue downhill on sagebrush-scented switchbacks, crossing the boundary to leave John Muir Wilderness. Stop to smell your last butterscotch-scented ponderosa pine as a series of zigzags leads you to the parking lot at Whitney Portal (8,365 feet). Public restrooms are directly across from the trailhead, while food, showers (fee), a pay phone, and the general store are to the right. The burger-and-fries combination is worth every cent! The general store is open daily in May and October from 9 a.m. to 6 p.m.; June and September from 8 a.m. to 8 p.m.; and July and August from 7 a.m. to 9 p.m.

PERMIT INFORMATION: *Permits that originate in the Inyo National Forest can be reserved by contacting the Wilderness Permit Reservation Office (351 Pacu Lane, Suite 200, Bishop, CA 93514), open 8 a.m. to 4:30 p.m. daily from June 1 to October 1 and Monday through Friday during the rest of the year. You can reserve over the phone at (760) 873-2483, by fax at (760) 873-2484, or by mail. You will need to provide the following information: name; address; daytime phone number; number of people in the party; method of travel (foot); number of stock (if applicable); start and end dates; entry and exit trailheads (Onion Valley entry,*

Whitney Portal exit); principal destination; credit-card number and expiration date, money order, or check for a nonrefundable $15-per-person processing fee.

If you are traveling south on US 395, you can pick up your permit at the White Mountain Ranger Station (798 North Main Street, Bishop, CA 93514). Office hours are 8 a.m. to 5 p.m.; (760) 873-2500.

If you are traveling north on US 395, you can pick up your permit in Lone Pine at the Eastern Sierra InterAgency Visitor Center (junction of US 395 and SR 136. Office hours are 8 a.m. to 5 p.m.; (760) 876-6200. About 60 percent of permits are reservable, the remainder are set aside for walk-in permits.

DIRECTIONS: ONION VALLEY TRAILHEAD—The closest town to the Onion Valley trailhead is Independence on US 395, 16 miles north of Lone Pine and 26 miles south of Big Pine. From Independence, drive west on Market Street for 13 miles. The road name eventually changes to Onion Valley Road, and the trailhead lies at its terminus (9,180 feet).

You can take public transit as far as Independence via Inyo Mono Transit's CREST bus, but you will need to walk or hitchhike the remaining 13 miles to the trailhead. The bus travels north on US 395 between Bishop and Reno via Mammoth Lakes on Tuesday, Thursday, and Friday, and south between Mammoth Lakes and Ridgecrest on Monday, Wednesday, and Friday. Independence lies 45 minutes south of Bishop. Rates and routes are subject to frequent change; call ahead for information and reservations at (760) 872-1901 or (800) 922-1930. More information can be found on the Web at www.county ofinyo.org/transit/CRESTpage.htm.

WHITNEY PORTAL TRAILHEAD—Whitney Portal lies 13 miles west of Lone Pine, off US 395, at the end of Whitney Portal Road. There is no public transit to the portal itself, but every car that leaves the parking lot goes through Lone Pine, so it's fairly easy to hitch a ride.

Inyo Mono Transit's CREST buses travel from Lone Pine south 1.5 hours to Ridgecrest and north to Bishop (1 hour) or Mammoth Lakes (2 hours). From Bishop, it's possible to transfer to another bus farther north to Reno. Rates and routes are subject to frequent change; call ahead for information and reservations at (760) 872-1901 or (800) 922-1930. More information can be found on the Web at www.countyofinyo.org/transit/CRESTpage.htm.

GPS coordinates	*Starting trailhead* ONION VALLEY
UTM zone (WGS84):	11S
Easting	0380432
Northing	4070625
Latitude	N 36°46'25.95"
Longitude	W 118°20'23.37"

GPS Trailhead Coordinates	*Ending trailhead* WHITNEY PORTAL
UTM zone (WGS84):	11S
Easting	0388918
Northing	4049743
Latitude	N 36°35'12.14"
Longitude	W 118°14'30.21"

CLOTHING
Synthetic shorts
Noncotton T-shirt
Sock liners
Socks
Underwear
Long-sleeve T-shirt
Long pants
Long underwear
Boots
Camp shoes
Fleece jacket
Down vest
Raincoat
Hat/gloves
Sun hat
Bandanna

EQUIPMENT
Tent or shelter
Sleeping bag
Sleeping pad
Thin plastic ground cover
    (doubles as a rain shelter)
Water filter
Stove
Fuel
Water bottle and/or hydration
    system

Duct tape (for emergency repairs
    and bandage adhesion)
Pot
Potholder
Spoon/fork
Dish
Mug
Sponge/biodegradable suds
Sunscreen/lip balm
Toothpaste
Toilet paper and plastic bag to
    pack it out
Trowel
Camera and spare batteries
GPS and spare batteries
Headlamp or flashlight
First-aid kit
Swiss Army knife
Collapsible water carrier
Bear can
Maps
Wilderness permit
ID/money
Garbage bag to cover pack in rain
Thin pillowcase
Cards/journal/book

Appendix B: First-aid Kit

A typical first-aid kit may contain more items than you might think necessary. These are just the basics. Prepackaged kits in waterproof bags (Atwater Carey and Adventure Medical make a variety of kits) are available. Even though there are quite a few items listed here, they pack down into a small space:

Ace bandages or Spenco joint wraps

Antibiotic ointment (Neosporin or the generic equivalent)

Aspirin or acetaminophen

Band-Aids

Benadryl or the generic equivalent, diphenhydramine (in case of allergic reactions)

Butterfly-closure bandages

Epinephrine in a prefilled syringe (for people known to have severe allergic reactions to such things as bee stings)

Gauze (one roll)

Gauze compress pads (a half-dozen 4- x 4-inch pads)

Hydrogen peroxide or iodine

Insect repellent

Matches or pocket lighter

Moleskin/Spenco "Second Skin"

Sunscreen

Whistle (it's more effective in signaling rescuers than your voice)

Appendix C: Contact Information

YOSEMITE NATIONAL PARK
P.O. Box 577
Yosemite National Park,
CA 95389
(209) 372-0200
www.nps.gov/yose

INYO NATIONAL FOREST
351 Pacu Lane
Suite 200
Bishop, CA 93514
(760) 873-2400
www.fs.fed.us/r5/inyo

SIERRA NATIONAL FOREST
1600 Tollhouse Road
Clovis, CA 93611
(559) 297-0706
www.fs.fed.us/r5/sierra

DEVILS POSTPILE NATIONAL MONUMENT
P.O. Box 3999
Mammoth Lakes, CA
93546
(760) 934-2289
www.nps.gov/depo

SEQUOIA AND KINGS CANYON NATIONAL PARKS
47050 Generals Highway
Three Rivers, CA 93271
(559) 565-3341
www.nps.gov/seki

PACIFIC CREST TRAIL ASSOCIATION
5325 Elkhorn Boulevard
PMB #256
Sacramento, CA 95842
(916) 349-2109
www.pcta.org/about_trail /muir/links.asp

SIERRA CLUB
85 Second Street
2nd Floor
San Francisco, CA 94105
(415) 977-5500
www.sierraclub.org

Index

About the Author

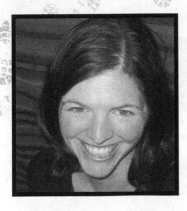

Kathleen Dodge first shouldered a backpack at the tender age of 10 when her dad forced her to walk around the neighborhood with a pack full of encyclopedias to prepare for her inaugural overnight outing in Yosemite. From the first heavily laden step, a love affair was born, and a thirst for backcountry adventure has led Kathleen to decades of starry nights in her native California. Kathleen toasted her 30th birthday from the top of Mount Whitney after completing the John Muir Trail for the first time, and she has returned every summer thereafter. A graduate of the University of California, Berkeley, Kathleen also spends her time leading hiking and biking trips around the globe, travel-writing, and planning her next adventure while holed up in Oakland and San Francisco cafes with great books.

DEAR CUSTOMERS AND FRIENDS,

SUPPORTING YOUR INTEREST IN OUTDOOR ADVENTURE, travel, and an active lifestyle is central to our operations, from the authors we choose to the locations we detail to the way we design our books. Menasha Ridge Press was incorporated in 1982 by a group of veteran outdoorsmen and professional outfitters. For 25 years now, we've specialized in creating books that benefit the outdoors enthusiast.

Almost immediately, Menasha Ridge Press earned a reputation for revolutionizing outdoors- and travel-guidebook publishing. For such activities as canoeing, kayaking, hiking, backpacking, and mountain biking, we established new standards of quality that transformed the whole genre, resulting in outdoor-recreation guides of great sophistication and solid content. Menasha Ridge continues to be outdoor publishing's greatest innovator.

The folks at Menasha Ridge Press are as at home on a white-water river or mountain trail as they are editing a manuscript. The books we build for you are the best they can be, because we're responding to your needs. Plus, we use and depend on them ourselves.

We look forward to seeing you on the river or the trail. If you'd like to contact us directly, join in at www.trekalong.com or visit us at www.menasharidge.com. We thank you for your interest in our books and the natural world around us all.

SAFE TRAVELS,

Bob Sehlinger

BOB SEHLINGER
PUBLISHER